TOUGH
Women Who Survived Cancer

TOUGH: Women Who Survived Cancer

Publisher's Note
This book portrays the contributors' experience with cancer, and the publisher's intent is not to provide medical advice with the material presented. If you are in need of treatment, psychological advice, or medical services please seek an experienced medical provider or health care professional.

Author's Note
The identities of some of the contributors in this collection have been disguised or composited to protect their privacy. Any errors in recollection of the events by the contributors are their own.

Published by:
Share Triumph Press, a division of AuthorpreneurLaunch LLC
4401 4 th Ave. #D3
Brooklyn, NY 11220
www.ShareTriumph.com

Editor: Sara Grace
Line Editor: Pamela Rafalow Grossman
Additional Copy: Dave Fischer
Cover Illustration: Tabi Walters
Cover Design: Matt Davies
Map Graphic Design and Kickstarter Design: Jeff Blum
Formatting: Eddie Knight
Publishing and Marketing Advice: Tom Swyers
Additional Marketing: Cem Hurturk
Interviewer and Story Collector: Marquina Iliev-Piselli
Kickstarter Video: Produced and Directed by Dennis Cahlo

ISBN 978-1-7330342-0-3 (Print)
ISBN 978-1-7330342-1-0 (Ebook)

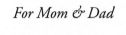

For Mom & Dad

TABLE OF CONTENTS

INTRODUCTION

The Women of Tough

by Marquina Iliev-Piselli

This book isn't about me. It's about the women I interviewed, whose stories made me fall in love with every one of them. Their guts and grit – and honesty – blows me away every time I read their essays. Still, I'll tell you the Cliff's Notes version of my story, because it introduces the inspiration and intent of TOUGH.

I'm Marquina – a mother, wife, digital marketer, breast cancer survivor, competitive air- guitarist, insufferable karaoke singer, and all-around goofball living in Brooklyn, NY. In September of 2015 I found a small lump in my right breast. Everyone said "It's nothing." But I ended up getting a mammogram, sonogram, and biopsy. It was something, all right. I was diagnosed in October of 2015, and chemotherapy started November 1. My last treatment was on Halloween of 2016, and I've been in remission for almost three years.

In the months after my diagnosis, I experienced uncertainty, sadness, anger, and pure fear. That fear caused me to retreat into myself. I didn't want to talk to anyone about my diagnosis, because it was too painful to relive with each retelling. Each time I would muster the courage to discuss what I was going through, I left the interaction feeling depleted and raw. At a certain point, I didn't want to talk, walk, smile, or leave my bed. I was short-tempered with my husband and son. I felt stalled. Stuck.

When I started chemo, I knew that to get through it, I needed to find something that could make going through treatment not sad anymore. I didn't want to sit for eight hours a day doing nothing and being afraid. I landed on what I called Glam Chemo. I was donated fabulous dresses, jewelry, wigs, and crowns. My friend Eden Di Bianco, a makeup artist, agreed to come in and do my makeup for some of my chemo sessions at NewYork-Presbyterian/Weill Cornell Medical Center. I put beautiful painted designs on my bald head. Casey Fatchett, the photographer who shot my wedding, took pictures of me looking…well, you can see for yourself if you Google "glam chemo" and *People* magazine, which did a piece on this project.

I didn't originally plan to go public with the pictures. They were for me, to turn my saddest days into my best ones. I wasn't getting chemo—no! I was in a photo shoot, smiling the whole time. It made the time fun. The next day, of course, I always felt terrible. But two days later, Casey would send me the pictures and I'd think, *Oh, yeah. Amazing!* I might have had a raging headache right then, but I'd see the photos and know: *Yeah, I can do this. It's okay. It's gonna be all right.*

Every couple of weeks I got dressed up and tried to make something special happen in those six to eight hours. It saved me. It saved my spirit. And it still is saving me, because now, I don't look back on that time with fear. Instead, I remember how my friends and family came together for me. My brother came, and we re-enacted some of our childhood photos, which was hilarious—me in a baby bib or a Mickey Mouse t-shirt. My best friend came, and a bunch of fellow air guitarists came (air guitar being another one of my life-saving creative passions). We did trust falls in the lobby, which was not sanctioned. We did it because that's what air guitarists do. We do spontaneous, very, very safe, mildly crazy things.

I made the best of chemotherapy that I possibly could. Glam Chemo isn't for everyone; but my experience made me wonder how other women got through it. It also made me want to encourage others to find *their* thing. It might be something they've always wanted to do but felt blocked from by fear or inertia. Or it might be something completely unknown to them until they discover it and take the first step. It might begin during treatment or after. The question is: What's that one thing that can save you from sinking into yourself and retreating from life? What can light you up, even in the worst times, and connect you to a community?

This line of thinking, along with my inability to find a book serving up a bunch of stories like this, lead me to create TOUGH. I went on an eight-month journey to find and interview women who had embraced creative pursuits or found otherwise inspiring ways to weather the emotional earthquake of cancer.

And I found them! Their stories are as diverse as they are: The women dove into writing, stand-up comedy, lip-synching, furniture restoration, quilting, you name it. Together with an editor and the women themselves, we turned their interviews into essays; and the result is a giant, inspiring, sometimes emotionally raw oral history of heroines. My hope is that through TOUGH, any reader can immediately surround herself with a circle of women who get it—and have wisdom to share.

Get ready for honest, inspiring, uplifting, rock-n-rolling, gut-wrenching, heart-pounding, chemo-brain-fueled tales about cancer and its aftermath.

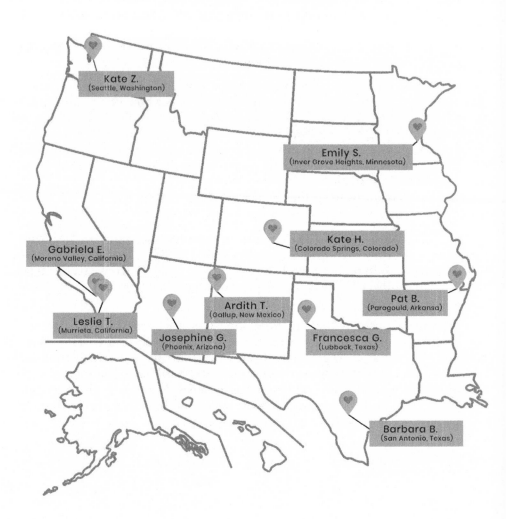

Kate Z.
(Seattle, Washington)

Emily S.
(Inver Grove Heights, Minnesota)

Kate H.
(Colorado Springs, Colorado)

Gabriela E.
(Moreno Valley, California)

Pat B.
(Paragould, Arkansa)

Ardith T.
(Gallup, New Mexico)

Leslie T.
(Murrieta, California)

Josephine G.
(Phoenix, Arizona)

Francesca G.
(Lubbock, Texas)

Barbara B.
(San Antonio, Texas)

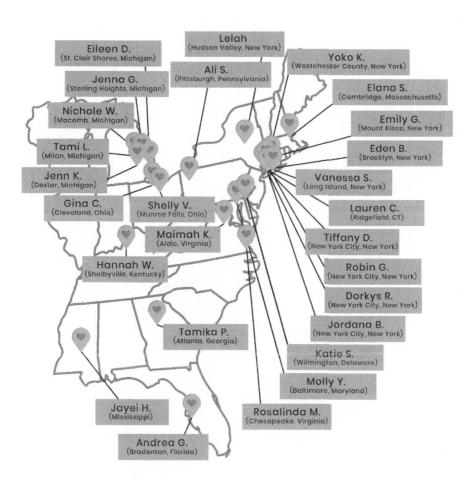

Eileen D.
(St. Clair Shores, Michigan)

Lelah
(Hudson Valley, New York)

Yoko K.
(Westchester County, New York)

Jenna G.
(Sterling Heights, Michigan)

Ali S.
(Pittsburgh, Pennsylvania)

Elana S.
(Cambridge, Massachusetts)

Nichole W.
(Macomb, Michigan)

Emily G.
(Mount Kisco, New York)

Tami L.
(Milan, Michigan)

Eden B.
(Brooklyn, New York)

Jenn K.
(Dexter, Michigan)

Vanessa S.
(Long Island, New York)

Gina C.
(Cleveland, Ohio)

Shelly V.
(Munroe Falls, Ohio)

Lauren C.
(Ridgefield, CT)

Maimah K.
(Aldie, Virginia)

Tiffany D.
(New York City, New York)

Hannah W.
(Shelbyville, Kentucky)

Robin G.
(New York City, New York)

Dorkys R.
(New York City, New York)

Jordana B.
(New York City, New York)

Tamika P.
(Atlanta, Georgia)

Katie S.
(Wilmington, Delaware)

Molly Y.
(Baltimore, Maryland)

Jayei H.
(Mississippi)

Rosalinda M.
(Chesapeake, Virginia)

Andrea G.
(Bradenton, Florida)

WEST & SOUTHWEST

Two Diagnoses & One Proposal

Name: Francesca Elizabeth Dials

Town: Lubbock, Texas

Diagnosis: Osteosarcoma in nasal cavity; myelodysplastic syndrome

Age at diagnosis: 25, then 28

Age now: 30

Before my first diagnosis, in 2014, I had just graduated from Texas Tech, a college here in Lubbock, and I was getting ready to move to Austin, Texas, with my best friend, Erica. I had been offered a management position at Torchy's Tacos. Lubbock had been my home for 25 years, so this was a big change. Austin is a great city, and I was really looking forward to a new career. Unfortunately, I was diagnosed a couple months after my move, so it was one quick change after another. After I was diagnosed, it was better for me to move back home.

The story started with me waking up one morning with an eye that was swollen almost shut. I went to a walk-in clinic, and they thought I had a staph infection. They told me, "You're going to be off of work a few days, but we'll give you a shot and put you on antibiotics, and you should be good."

The next day, I woke up with a debilitating migraine. Erica took me to Saint David's for a CT scan, at the clinic's recommendation. Afterward we were sitting in the exam room waiting for results—laughing, joking, and not really thinking anything of it. Then all of a sudden I looked at her and just asked, "What if it's bad?" She was confused—"What?" And I said, "What if something's wrong? What if there's something on the scan that's bad? What if it comes back that something's wrong?" She told me I was just freaking out.

BEST ADVICE: My best friend constantly told me to "rock the bald." I had a wig on, and she was like, "Just rip the wig off." It was so hot, and she said, "Rip it off, just take it off. Put it in your purse." I took it off, and it was literally the most freeing, just-didn't-care experience. That is one thing I always try to remember: Rock the bald. And not just the bald—rock the life. Whatever is placed in front of you, rock it, and don't let it hold you back. We are given one chance, one opportunity, so make it freaking awesome!

Ten minutes later, a doctor walked in, looked at me, and said, "You have a tumor in your sinus cavity. We need to do another scan. An ENT will be in to see you shortly." Then he walked out. He couldn't have had a worse delivery. I immediately started crying. Erica ran over to the exam table and hugged me while we decided who to call first. My dad? My mom? I didn't know how I was going to tell them.

Within a couple of days, I had a biopsy. We arranged for those results to go directly to my parents, and I went home to Lubbock to wait. Several days later, I walked into my parents' kitchen after having been out. I already knew something was up, because my mom had texted that I should come home. They were both standing there with my aunt, who is an RN; the fact that she had come was not a good sign. My aunt gave me a hug, and they said, "So he called, and it is cancerous." I was in shock. I remember my mom crying and my aunt telling me to sit down because I had lost all color in my face. I was just like, "What now?"

Osteosarcoma is a pretty aggressive cancer, and because of where mine was, the doctors wanted to start chemo right away. We found a top-notch neurologist in San Antonio and basically stalked him until he accepted me as a patient. I also had a full oncology team. I did the same protocol that they do for people who have osteosarcoma in a leg or an arm—usually teenagers. Unfortunately, some of the people have to lose part of a limb. Obviously, in my case, I couldn't lose my head, so my regimen was intense. I think I got three times the normal dose that they give teenagers, and my treatment included the chemo drug that people call the "red devil."

By the second day, I was definitely sick. I had the first two chemo rounds in San Antonio and then shifted to doing it outpatient in Lubbock. Having more family around made it easier. Unfortunately, after my third round, I had a seizure when I got home. They put me on seizure medication, and my last round before surgery was inpatient again. I went back down to San Antonio, and my surgery was on June 29. It was a 13-hour surgery. The ENT went through my nose, the neurologist cut open my head, and they met up and removed the tumor. They actually ended up having to take 36 tissue samples before they got a negative read on the margins. I obviously don't remember much of that day, except that as they were rolling me to the back, I threw the peace sign to my family when they were out of my view. I was glad they couldn't see my tears.

After that, I healed for a couple months and got my strength up. Then I did post-op chemo from October to February, all inpatient. Once May came around I was able to move back to Austin, where Erica was waiting for my return.

Prior to graduation and the big move, I had met my now-fiancé, Knowe, in Lubbock, and we'd become really good friends. We started dating during my treatment, in December of 2014. When you don't have your hair, you're not feeling like yourself. But he never saw me any differently. He stuck around through such difficult times, times when I made it clear to him that he didn't have to. I told him, "I don't want you to feel like you have to stay because I'm sick." He reminded me often, "If I was going to go, I would have gone." The thing is, I know him and I know his personality, and that's a fact.

If we were going to break up, if he were going to go his own direction, he would have done it.

I moved back to Austin in May 2015, after being in remission for a few months. I started my job as an hourly supervisor, so that I would have a designated amount of hours and could ease back in. (As a manager, your hours can be very long.) That worked well, so I got back into my management position. I went to San Antonio for evaluation every three months for the first couple of years, and everything checked out. Knowe and I were still dating, doing the whole long-distance thing. Everything was going really well.

In March 2017, I went for my 3-month scan and they noticed that the goiter in my thyroid, which I'd always had, looked like maybe it had grown. They got me in with an endocrinologist, who was actually going to do a biopsy that day. As I was filling out paperwork, the doctor came in and said, "I think you need to call your doctor. Your platelet and hemoglobin levels are extremely low." She didn't want to cut even a little slit in my neck to do a biopsy because she was afraid of any kind of blood loss or infection.

My oncologist in San Antonio immediately set me up for a bone marrow aspiration— which is so much fun, let me tell you. Then I waited more than a week. When my oncologist finally called me with results, he says, "We have some news. Your dad is on the line with us."

As soon as he said that, I knew: *Here we go again.* He told me that the scan showed that two of my chromosomes had bonded together—and it's very uncommon to see this in the two that had. I had MDS—myelodysplastic syndrome—which is similar to and treated the same way as leukemia.

I thought, *You've got to be kidding me.* My second diagnosis was almost exactly three years after my first diagnosis, to the day. It was almost creepy. "The doctor said, "We're going to have to do more chemo, and you're eventually going to need a stem cell transplant." His immediate recommendation was for me to go to M.D. Anderson, the massive cancer center in Houston. They treat all kinds of cancers, but they're very well-known for treating blood cancers, which is what I had. He didn't suggest any other options.

I told Torchy's once again, and again they were sad for me. This time around, they applied the Family Medical Leave Act, which guaranteed me paychecks and insurance for three months. After that, I had to get my own insurance, because I technically was not working for them anymore. But the FMLA bought me time to research insurance before making a decision.

In Houston, I ended up doing two rounds of chemo outpatient and then a third round in the hospital. The goal of the third round was to completely demolish my immune system so that I could rebuild from donor cells. Donors can be found in the registry, but if a sibling is available, they like to test them first. My brother immediately told M.D. Anderson to send him a kit. His blood sample showed he was 100% my perfect match. It was pretty cool that my brother graciously gave me eight million of his cells. I love to tell people that my brother saved my life.

When I had cancer the first time, he was younger, and it was a lot for him to handle. He didn't always want to come and visit me in the hospital, and I can understand that. Hospitals are sucky. I was never mad at him. But this time around, he felt really good about being able to be there for me in a big way. Meanwhile, I had to sit back and accept that my younger brother was going to take care of me. Our roles were reversed.

My transplant was on June 6. I had a PICC line. They had divided his cells into these eight little baggies. They would hook one up, and it would take maybe five minutes for it to run. I watched them go into my body. Then they would wait an hour and do another one.

I can't smell anymore, because the surgery to remove the tumor from my nasal cavity destroyed my sense of smell. But apparently you smell like a tomato when you're having this transplant. Every nurse would walk by my room, smell the tomato, and poke their head in to say, "Oh, happy birthday." I was like, "Happy birthday? It's not my birthday." They explained that getting a new immune system is kind of like being born again.

After the transplant I was in the hospital for almost 30 days, constrained to one floor because I still didn't have a functioning immune system. It was extremely trying, even though I had visitors. Most of the time, I walked circles. They force you to walk multiple times a day, and they make it a game by giving you stickers every time you do. You get to hang the stickers on your door. It made my door look exciting and fun. Actually, I probably walked more than I ever had in my entire life. I had my Fitbit on, counting my steps. Knowe bought it for me.

Recovering from the transplant was difficult and painful. It changed my skin. I looked like I had chemo burn all over my body, almost like the top layer of my skin died with the transplant. It was very hard to look at myself. Thankfully, Knowe was always so sweet. I would say, "I feel really ugly, and I hate it," and I'd still know he never looked at me any differently. Some people can't handle it. He was there the entire time.

He proposed three days after my transplant, when I literally was at my worst. It was awful. I had a symptom that every transplant patient gets: When I swallowed, it felt like knives. It lasted like two weeks. I was getting my meds through an IV because I couldn't swallow pills. I was laying there, feeling like death. Knowe came over and laid in bed with me. He looked at me and said, "I'm sorry." I asked him what he was sorry about, and he started to get teary eyed. "It's not fair that you're going through this again. I'm just sorry that you're here. I'm sorry that we're here." I told him, "You know, I always told myself when I went through it the first time, if it happens again, there will be a reason. I might not understand it, but I'm just going to have to figure it out." He said, "I know, but right now I just don't see a legitimate reason." Then he just started to ramble, but in a cute way. He said, "I've been trying to plan it, but things just keep happening. I've been talking to people, and I asked your dad, and your dad was like, 'No, you'll just know. You have to ask her. It doesn't need to be this big set up. That's not Franki's personality.'"

I started tearing up because I knew what was about to happen. He said, "I've been trying to do this big fancy thing, and it just seems like it's just not right, it's just not you. I feel it, and I'm just going to ask you. I know this isn't the best time, and you're in this terrible place, but I just know I want you to be my wife, and I don't care what comes our way from here. We can get through it. I don't even have a ring yet, but I knew I needed to do it now." I was bawling and nodding my head yes. I said, "I don't care that you don't have a ring." It was perfect!

We have faced a lot of challenges, and recently there has been another one. My first cancer was so aggressive that there was no question about stopping for fertility planning. The second time, we discussed freezing my eggs, but my platelets were too low to do it. Now, I would like to have babies. Knowe has a daughter from a previous long-term relationship, Kayla. She's great, and I love her. I can't wait to be a stepmom, but I'd also like to have biological children. At this point, they aren't sure if I'll be able to produce my own eggs, but they tell me I'll be able to carry a baby. It may not be how I originally thought it would happen, but that was nice to hear. The doctor also told me, "Your body can all of a sudden decide that it wants to start working the way it's supposed to be working." You just never really know. We're going to keep our fingers crossed and just keep going. We've talked about it. If it doesn't happen, there are many children that need parents, and I will happily bring them into my home.

Recently wedding planning has taken over everything, but I'm planning to go back to school for massage therapy, with a focus on cancer patients, as a way to give back. Many doctors are trying to implement massage therapy to help flush out the lymphatic system.

Today, I'm embracing the changes that I've seen in myself. I've always been very open and social. I've never been afraid to talk to people or make friends. But there were other parts of me that I was holding back, and I think cancer helped me express those things. I've always tried to be the person who is strong for everybody else. Cancer helped me open up a more vulnerable side of myself, which I was really fearful of letting people see. Extremely fearful, actually. To let that wall down and be able to show such a vulnerable side of me was something I had to work on. Still, to this day.

I sit here and think about all that's happened. I still think, "I went through it once, and then it was put in my path again a second time. There is reasoning behind it." I still don't think I have fully come to grasp what that might be. But I think there's something big in my future, and I'm excited about it, whatever it is.

Making Peace with a
Double Mastectomy

Name: Kate Zickel

Town: Seattle, Washington

Diagnosis: Breast cancer; stage 3; ER+, PR+; HER2-; invasive ductal carcinoma plus DCIS

Age at diagnosis: 30

Age now: 31

My friends in college used to joke that I was like a moth in a room full of Bunsen burners, flitting from one thing to the next, always happy and excited about the next thing. Since my diagnosis, that has changed. What makes me happiest now are the people in my life, whether it's someone special I meet once who makes an impact or someone who has been holding my hand the whole time. Those connections are what really matter to me. It's actually better than before, because it's a joy that's more grounded, reliable, and lasting.

Right before my diagnosis, I told anybody in my family who asked how I was doing that "Life is boring, but in a good way." There wasn't much going on, which was nice because in the years before there had been a lot of moving, a lot of ups and downs and job changes. But the previous couple years had been pretty relaxed

WORST ADVICE: About a week after I was diagnosed, some acquaintances—I wouldn't call them friends—said that they had "a word from the Lord" for me and invited me over to their house to talk. Not thinking too much about it, I drove 45 minutes to their house by myself. When I got there, it turned out that their words from the Lord were "rebellion and insolence." They said that even though God doesn't send us things like cancer, sometimes He uses them to make us better people and cure us of things like rebellion and insolence. That wasn't really advice, but it was probably the worst thing anyone's ever said to me in all of this—trying to convince me that somehow cancer was connected to a personal character flaw.

Then one day my husband found a lump the size of a marble near my left nipple. I received my diagnosis on September 21, 2017. The same day, a group of close friends came to our place. We all talked and prayed and discussed what our mentality was going to be like in the times ahead, how I could keep a positive attitude and best take care of myself—which was so great, because it really set the stage for everything that's happened since then. It was also where I established the idea of intense transparency and honesty around my experience.

I have a very strong religious faith, but I also have a strong faith in the people around me. My relationships are very important to me. The one thing at the very beginning that I remember being afraid of was that my relationship with my husband would change. It has, very much—but in a good way. Brian and I have learned to be honest, regardless of how painful it is. I am more direct with him than I used to be and have learned to ask for help when I need it. But in the beginning, I was afraid that things would change and that we wouldn't be able to connect or relate to each other the way we used to.

My approach to fear in general has always been the same: Be honest, be straightforward, talk about it, and stick to the belief that no matter what else changes, the God that I know is still the same. My faith is different now, because it's no longer connected to circumstance. Love is there even when joy and happiness have disappeared—especially then. I had to give up the idea that every dark moment has a silver lining. Sometimes it doesn't. But that's when love gets real.

The day after I was diagnosed, I went into work a little bit early to tell my boss. I said, "Yesterday I was diagnosed with breast cancer, and I just wanted you to know." As with my friends, I wanted to be very open and honest about all of it right away. I had no idea how offices handle things like cancer treatment. It's not something that you ask in an interview.

He was very sympathetic and even connected me with another woman who'd had breast cancer in our office 10 years ago. An hour later I got a call from HR, they set up an appointment to talk with me. Then I pulled the four girls I'm closest to in my office into a little room and said, "Look, I want you guys to know first." They were all really nice about it. Then I went out to the main office area and called out to the whole room. "All right, guys, I'm just going to make this simple. I'm going to make an announcement," I said. I figured it was easier than telling 15 people individually.

"This is super awkward, but I just wanted everybody to know that I was diagnosed with breast cancer yesterday. Please feel free to make as many death and boob jokes as you want over the next several months, because I think they're funny and I'm going to need them." The first thing one of my male coworkers said was, "I thought you were going to tell us all you were pregnant!" I started to laugh and said, "Well, not exactly." Looking back, it cracks me up, because ultimately treatment has taken up about the same amount of time as a pregnancy. Everybody took it really well.

I made a Facebook page that day too. It's called Kate Kicks Cancer (Facebook.com/KateKicksItToCancer). When I made the page, Facebook sent me an alert that said, "There's already a page called Kate Kicks Cancer. Do you need to go to that page?" I immediately wondered who the other Kate Kicks Cancer was, and I went to her page. Her name is Kate Larkin, and she has stage 4 disease, with some serious complications.

A few days later, I Facebook messaged her: "Hey, I know you might think this is super weird or creepy, but I found your page because my name's also Kate, and I'm kicking cancer too." We started Facebook messaging. After a month of that, we exchanged phone numbers. I called her on the way home one day, and we talked for two hours. We have talked on the phone at least once a week for about two hours ever since. Over Memorial Day last month, she flew out to visit me, and we went to the beach together for four days. We had never met before. It was the craziest thing, and we had the best time.

I started chemo about a month after diagnosis, October 25th. I did four rounds of Adriamycin and Cytoxan, and then four rounds of Taxol. It was dose-dense, every other week. My clinic offered cold capping, but it wasn't worth it to me to sit with ice on my head for three hours and pay $3,000 to keep my hair. For some people that's important, but I knew knew from the beginning that going bald was not my biggest fear. I barely wore makeup, although I wear more now. When your physical appearance falls completely apart, you find ways to keep it up where you can.

I'm the oldest of six kids, and I have always had a hard time asking for help, accepting help, or admitting when I need help. Once I got sick, I couldn't avoid it. I had to and wanted to accept help. But it was still a process of learning to say, "Oh, I need help. Can you do this for me?" I've gotten much better at it than I used to be. My friend Kara Tippets, who died from breast cancer that spread to her brain, talked a lot about how suffering is often an unexpected way that people can learn to love you and you can learn to accept love. That's what happened to Kara. She had a lot of people surrounding her and loving her, in ways that she didn't even know were possible, and I've had that too.

Since I was diagnosed, people have surrounded me with love in ways that I never would have thought of or imagined. When I learned it would be helpful to have someone with me at chemo, my husband sent an email to all of my local friends and said, "Hey, Kate's starting chemo. Here's her schedule. Could people please sign up to take her and drive her home?" I think it maybe took a couple of hours and all the slots were gone. People were actually fighting over slots.

My sister flew out and surprised me for my surgery. My coworkers pooled together to make me huge gift bags, and they also provided the majority of my meals during chemotherapy. I had people who emailed me when our company switched HSA plans, meaning I had to pay medical bills out of pocket for about a month and a half, saying, "If you need help paying your medical bills while this transition happens, we are here for you." I've had patient navigators who've never even met me stay on the phone with me for two and a half hours answering all of my questions, allaying all of my fears.

My sister-in-law and my husband conspired and sent out an APB to everyone I know— family, Facebook friends, old church friends, everybody— and said, "We're putting together chemo bags for Kate. If you want to send something, here's the address." There were 250 contributors, and each round of chemo I got a gift bag full of stuff that people had sent just to make me feel better that day. The gifts filled eight tote-sized shopping bags—coloring books, hard candies, funny wigs, lotions, pillows, comic books. You name it, it was in the bags. Every round of chemo, whoever was taking me to chemo that day would show up with one of these bags, and then somewhere during the hours of chemo, we'd open it together. My nieces and nephews all wrote me little notes. My favorite part about these bags wasn't even so much what was in them, but just being amazed at how many people had contributed and how much thought had gone into the gifts.

BEST ADVICE: When I first was diagnosed, I went to one of the Facebook groups and said, "What's the one thing you'd do differently?" I got 123 comments on that. An answer I saw a lot was, "I'd wait to make important life decisions until everything was over."

Of everything that happened to me during my recovery process, the most intense time was the period of almost eight weeks after chemo when I had to decide whether to have the mastectomy. It was an incredibly difficult and emotionally intense period for me, maybe only second to when my parents split up.

From the very beginning, I had said I wanted to avoid surgery and was told that the size of my tumors made that unlikely. I had very attractive size-D breasts that to me had always been my favorite physical thing about myself. From the second I got cancer, if I knew your first and last name and you were a woman and you wanted to see my boobs or find out what a tumor felt like in your boob, you could touch my boobs. I would show you. I showed them to one close friend of mine in a restaurant bathroom, and she said, "Man, you have plastic-surgeon-perfect tits." It was really hard for me to let that part of myself go. It took months of back-and-forth and research and medical pros and cons. I met with my poor surgeon four times to have him basically tell me, over and over and over again, that a double mastectomy was the best option to prevent recurrence and avoid additional radiation. He explained that multifocal, multicentric tumors can be more dangerous considering my age and my genetic mutations.

Four or five days before my surgery, I called those same friends who had come the first night. We all got together and had dinner and talked and prayed. I kept saying, "I don't know what to do." My friend Mary said, "You keep saying that, but the way you're presenting this to us it sounds like you've already decided." That was really all I needed—someone to help me acknowledge what I was thinking. All I could see was the dilemma, having to choose between two bad options.

From the beginning, Brian and I had been guided by the words of a friend: "Go where the peace is." Up until surgery, the peace and the medical recommendations had gone hand-in-hand. It wasn't difficult. But surgery was forcing me to lose something important to me, and I wasn't ready to let go. Chemo had worked so well that my tumors were no longer physically visible, which is almost unheard of (happens in less than 5% of cases). Brian and I both asked my surgeon, "Why would we need to remove completely healthy breast tissue?" The IDC was completely gone. But the chemo I had only kills the IDC. The DCIS was still there, in the right breast, which was the reason for the double mastectomy.

Ultimately, I had to stop trying to make the decision using data and statistics, trying to make the right medical choice. I couldn't decide that way. It had to be a decision of faith. I had to chose to listen to the doctors and believe that regardless of where things went, it was going to be OK. It wasn't going to be end of the world. And once I did the surgery, honestly, I did feel totally at peace with it. Although the reconstruction process was painful, I'm happy with the results. They healed up very quickly, and they look great.

Throughout my treatment, I documented things in short videos and shared them on Facebook. I made several with my plastic surgeon. At some point I realized I could piece this all together to make a coherent story.

I've always loved stories. I had worked as both a radio and film producer for a long time. So I had that background, but the videos were also inspired by my friend Kara (https://www.mundanefaithfulness.com/), who passed away. She had done videos when she was sick. They made a profound impact on my life, on the way that I view suffering and how I see my relationships with other people. Thanks to Kara, it was really important to me from the beginning to be very honest with the people in my life about what I was going through. I didn't want to have to put a smiley, happy face on everything. At the same time, I believed that even when suffering, it was possible to have a positive attitude.

Starting with my meeting Kate Larkin, Facebook and the whole storytelling platform that is social media have really brought a lot of people together, in a way that I wasn't expecting at all. It's been really, really positive. I met a woman the other night at a breast cancer event and we were talking about my plastic surgeon. She goes, "Oh my god, you're Kate. I saw your video. I know who you are." I was just floored. She knew all of these things about my story, because she had watched my video on my plastic surgeon's page and then gone to my page. Part of the reason for my honesty and transparency in sharing these videos is that hopefully if somebody else has to deal with this crap, there's something there to make it feel a little more manageable.

Finding Myself, Single After Cancer

Name: Josephine Guzman

Town: Phoenix, Arizona

Diagnosis: Breast cancer; stage 3; ER-, PR-, HER2- ("triple negative"); BRCA1+

Age at diagnosis: 37

Age now: 40

I was working full-time in the health insurance field, as a prior-authorization representative handling referrals for providers, when I was diagnosed. My three kids were 16, 9, and 4. I was also taking care of my mom, who had been diagnosed with breast cancer herself two months before. This was her second time; her first had been 10 years earlier.

It was taking care of her that led me to do a self-exam. I felt the lump and immediately knew. I pinched around it because it was on the upper part of my chest, and I was like, "No, this is totally weird." I was in so much shock. I went to my mom and sister and said, "Look, this is weird, right?" And right after that I started looking for a new primary-care doctor, because I didn't have one at that time.

When my mom had cancer the first time, I only went to maybe two of her appointments. I didn't know much about cancer, and she didn't make a big deal about it. The second time around, it scared us both, especially since we were both diagnosed around the same time. Thankfully, being in the medical field, I've had front- and back-office experience. So I knew how to read medical records, schedule appointments, and get things done.

WORST ADVICE: "Get over it. You don't have cancer anymore. It's nothing. It'll pass." I don't think people know that it never passes. I've been cancer-free since December 2016, when I had my double mastectomy; however, I'm still living with the side effects of cancer.

My mom's mom was diagnosed with breast cancer while I was pregnant with my youngest son. Cancer runs in my dad's side of the family, my mom's side of the family, and both of her parents' sides of the family. My mom chose not to get tested for BRCA when she was first diagnosed. I wanted all the tests. I always tried to prepare for this day. I always got the cancer insurance, cancer benefits from work—just in case, God forbid, this happened. However, I found out after I got diagnosed that for some reason, through open enrollment, I had never finalized the paperwork for that benefit. One missed signature and a lack of communication caused me not to have that backup plan, which could have been a tremendous help.

I found the lump in mid-April. By the time I'd seen my primary-care doctor, it was the beginning of May. Immediately they said, "Let's do a mammogram." By the end of May, I had my biopsy. I told the doctor, "I don't want to come in for results. I just want you to tell me immediately." So they told me over the phone, while I was at work in a training class. I had to take it all in when she said, "Your results came back positive. We'll need you to choose your doctors and let us know what you want to do." And I said, "So I have cancer? ... Are you sure?" I was in total disbelief. She confirmed and said, "We need to start making the next steps." I had just gone through everything with my mom, setting up her surgeon, her oncologist, and her radiation oncologist, so for me it was simple. I went to all the same doctors. That way, we would be together. It was kind of like we became each other's caregiver at that point. We were close before, but this brought us ten thousand times closer.

She started chemo before me, in early June, and then I started right before the Fourth of July. We had the same treatment: Two types of chemo, Adriamycin and Cytoxan, for four rounds, once every two weeks; and then a third chemo, Taxol, weekly for 12 weeks.

During chemo, we just talked. The nurses were so nice—they used to sit us across from each other. Sometimes we listened to music and watched movies on our Ipads, but for the most part we just chit-chatted. Whoever finished first would sit by the other until she finished. A lot of people thought it was crazy that we were there together, both as patients, because I was 37 and my mom was 58.

They told me I was stage 2 at first, but when I got to radiation, I found that it was stage 3A. My mom at first was put at stage 3, but it turned out to be stage 4. We found that out at the end of her treatment.

I had the BRCA1 gene mutation, and the cancer was triple negative, which is an aggressive form. The lump when I found it was the size of a small marble. By the time I went to have chemo, a month or so later, it was huge. It filled up my whole breast. The first time I met with my oncologist, I had decided on a double mastectomy and a hysterectomy. With the BRCA1 mutation, you're at high risk of breast cancer, ovarian cancer, and pancreatic cancer. I made the choice to just get everything I could removed after radiation. It was a very easy choice. I told myself the day I was diagnosed, "My mom has cancer. I know I don't want it again. If it came back for her twice, why would I keep my breasts?"

Six weeks after getting my mastectomies and implants, I started radiation, daily except for the weekends. Three months after I finished radiation, I found that it was hard to rotate my arm, and I started getting a lot of pain in my upper chest. My implant started shifting on the right side, where I had been radiated, and the skin got tight. I ended up going in to my doctor. Imaging showed that I had a capsule forming around my right implant. They sent me to physical therapy, and that's when I got diagnosed with lymphedema, which never goes away.

As far as the shifted implant, I had to wait a year from the last time I had radiation to deal with it—so after March, I had my appointment. The implant had shifted so much at that point that it was literally under my collarbone and the right side of my armpit. I had to wear a mastectomy bra with a prosthetic to make my breasts look even. I felt so embarrassed, because I had to go through all this change, and then I was waiting, waiting, waiting, like, "When can I fix this?" Finally they said I could replace the implants and do a DIEP-flap surgery to reconstruct both breasts.

At the time I had been laid off, so I had to wait some more. Then I found a great permanent job with a great company, built up my vacation time, and just had my surgery yesterday. The surgery was actually only an hour and a half for a capsulectomy with replacement of implant. In the end, I did not do a full DIEP-flap reconstruction. Hopefully it's back in place where it belongs and won't get damaged again. They warned me that radiation can still change your body years later.

During my treatment, I lost my relationship of four and a half years. I hear it happens with a lot of cancer survivors. Some relationships can't withstand the trauma. I was diagnosed with depression and anxiety, and I had a really short fuse due to the hormonal changes after my hysterectomy. It was a really hard situation. At the same time, I have tried to stay strong, smile, and just do what I've got to do and live my life.

We separated in June, and I came to live with my younger brother and his family. It was a big transition. I love my job. It's crazy to say, but work is my happy place. I'm a concierge navigator for a great organization. My role is to work with insurance companies, patients, and doctors, helping to provide care-coordination resources for chronic diseases, and guiding patients along their way. It feels really good to give back. I can help make sure no one experiences what I did—losing out on a benefit because they didn't sign a form.

I work 9:30 to 6:00 every day. And every day I tell myself, "I want to get my own place and get back on my feet." I decided to get a second job to push things along. Tonight I have orientation to work as a cashier. I'm very, very busy. I take my kids back and forth to their dad's. I still have doctor appointments. I see my oncologist—and my endocrinologist, because I'm hypothyroid, too. That's another battle. I'm up every day at 6 a.m., seven days a week. I go to sleep at 11 p.m. so I can spend time with my kids, then take my oldest son to his father's.

I've started going back to church, just trying to find myself over these past couple months. There's no way to avoid the fear that I have in my mind. To me it sucks, because I feel most people don't get me. They don't get me because they haven't gone through it. I have fear every day, with every pain—"Is the cancer coming back?" However, I try to overcome it by keeping myself busy and addressing things with the doctor. I use meditation and music to get my mind off the fear of recurrence. These are things that I know we all do as breast cancer survivors.

Talking to other women cancer survivors of all kinds has really helped me. So did educating myself about cancer. In July 2017, I flew out to Boston after signing up to become a young advocate for Living Beyond Breast Cancer. I met 15 amazing women, of all ages. I'm still friends with them today on Facebook, and we share the same fears and the same issues. We reach out to each other when we have questions. A lot of women, unfortunately, have had recurrences, so we talk about it. We're able to ask, "Hey, what does this mean? Have you had this? Has this happened to you?"

And I'm in other groups, like a triple-negative group for women who have my same exact diagnosis, and people who are BRCA positive. I go to nonprofits here locally, and I keep in touch with local single moms or local moms affected by all kinds of cancer, not just breast cancer. We try to get together monthly, just to talk to each other, help each other, and educate each other. Some of them are stage 4, and we try to be each other's support. Some don't have family or friends, or their families are out of town. I'm fortunate to have all my family here, but you can still feel lonely.

My joy now, besides my job, is spending time with my friends and family as much as I can. I try to educate my family as well about our risks. My son just turned 18, so I let him know he can get tested. My goal is to travel more. With this cancer journey I went to Boston, Maui, and the Grand Canyon. I'd never done that before. I'm taking joy in trying to find myself, and traveling, and doing different things I'd never thought about doing. I don't wait. I try to live every day to the fullest. I find joy in meeting all these women and men who have been diagnosed and spending time with them.

Self-Portraits in a Dark & Messy Medium

· ·

Name: Kathryn Hust

Town: Colorado Springs, Colorado

Diagnosis: Breast cancer; stage 2; ER+, PR+, HER2+ ("triple positive")

Age at diagnosis: 36

Age now: 39

The summer before I was diagnosed, I knew change was coming. I had lived in a small town in Northern Michigan for about nine years and had always wrestled with my place there. Uncertain of our plans, my husband and I planned a little sabbatical of traveling with our family as we figured out our next step. Part of preparing for this included dentist and doctor appointments while we were still covered by insurance. My doctor appointment was the last one. That's when I discovered a lump—and it was clear that we wouldn't be gallivanting off as we'd thought.

In less than thirty days, we'd become jobless and homeless, and I'd been diagnosed with cancer. It was like a full stop. Through the years and all my prayers asking, "What do you have next for me?" I never pictured sickness as the answer. Yet because we were already in a state of transition, we were free to move wherever we needed to, and my husband was available to be my caregiver.

I've never been a disciplined journaler, even with advice and encouragement from others. I'm an artist, a visual person. Images and moments stick with me more than words. When I was diagnosed with breast cancer, things were happening so fast around me, good things and hard things, and I wanted a way to remember them. I began to write these moments and blessings down on little paper "leaves" that I eventually put together to make a wreath. I have it framed and hung in my bedroom, next to the door. Every time I walk by it, I remember the events and notable moments during this journey—the things that sustained me and words that encouraged me.

More than nine years in a small town had produced some really tight

BEST ADVICE: It came from my oncologist, who said, "Your body is fearfully and wonderfully made, and it's stronger than the cancer cells. Cancer cells are weak, but your body is strong." I feel like that drove home that while I might be sick from the medication, it was killing the weak cells. You'll lose some of the good cells, but they'll regenerate. The good ones are strong.

relationships, and leaving was harder than I'd expected. The love and generosity from people at my husband's work, our church, and the school district showed itself in many ways, including their throwing us a fundraiser. Initially, I felt guilty; the town as a whole had many needs and many residents in poverty. We had a savings account. I didn't want to take from them. Yet I learned that sometimes the best gift is accepting whatever others offer. Little acts added together make a big impact. I had been an art teacher, and the students from kindergarten through 12th grade, along with friends from the community, created pieces of artwork and donated crafts, jams, and quilts for a silent auction. It was so sweet to see friends of mine who didn't necessarily know each other working together, using their strengths to make this amazing event happen. Somebody organized all the auction donations. Someone organized a pancake dinner and volunteers to cook. Another made unique table decorations and placemats from young students' drawings. Somebody else made "Team Kate" bracelets that ended up being worn around the community. My proudest moment was when students who had donated artwork came up to me at the event, excitedly asking, "Did you see my painting sold? Did you see how much it sold for?" These are kids who don't have a lot of people saying encouraging things in their lives, and they felt like they'd contributed in such a big way—and they had. It was one thing for me to say "You're so talented," but now they got to see that others valued what they made. All together they all raised almost $12,000. This was the exact amount needed to cover my insurance for the year. My medical bills were extensive—and completely covered by this event.

My sister had recently bought a large house outside of Ann Arbor, and she generously invited us to live with her. She had already planned on storing our furniture and watching our dog while we traveled on our sabbatical, so what was four more people? She was in her own season of transition, expecting her first child. Our moving in marked the beginning of the most unexpected and sweetest nine-month season. Our husbands bonded, and we reconnected; I got to know my sister as an adult. Watching her become a mother and loving on my new baby niece were precious. Our daughters thrived with extra family around and always had someone home when they came back from school. My husband, Andy, was a caregiver to all of us. Those months were so rich with love and family when they could've been awful. I left a community that I had loved and cherished. I'd never planned on returning to live in my childhood town, but I would make the same decision again. It gave me a new sense of home.

After surgery, I immediately started six months of chemotherapy. You can only binge watch so much Netflix, so I started taking a portrait-drawing class in Ann Arbor. I had once owned a pottery business, but that art form was too messy and physically strenuous during this time. I'd always loved drawing but was not confident in portraits, especially of myself. Some people in the class painted, while I worked mostly in charcoal on gray paper. The medium was a little like the season I was in, dark and messy. I ended up making 16 portraits of myself, one for every round of chemotherapy. I put on 30 pounds when I was going through treatment, from the hormonal changes and the medicine. I look at the portraits today and *don't* feel like they look like me, because they really don't look like me.

Drawing became my much-needed emotional release valve. Early on, my doctor had said to me, "I don't want you to bottle up negative feelings. You're always so positive, so upbeat when you come here," and I replied, "I just haven't had them yet. I haven't had anger issues." Well, one day, I went to the doctor's office for my scheduled appointment. I went to my blood draw, and then I went to go see the oncologist. I was sitting there...and sitting there...and sitting there in the waiting room. It was about an hour past my appointment time, and I was just like, "What the heck? I have an appointment. This is why you make appointments—so that when you get there, they know you're coming, and you don't have to sit here and wait." The longer I sat, the more frustrated I got. It became this symbolic turning point for me: My whole life is already on hold, and now you're asking me to sit here and wait even more?

When I finally got into an exam room, I had a new nurse. When you go to cancer treatment, you get used to seeing the same nurses, doctors, and staff on a regular basis. At some point there is a connection, a relationship that builds. There is also what my husband and I joke about as "the sympathy hug," which is frequently exchanged around cancer patients. So this new girl came in, doing her job, but acting like we'd had a previous encounter. I was still fuming when she leaned over to give me a hug. Sensing my coldness, she said, "Is there anything else that I can do for you?" I'm usually a very kind and polite person, but I had had enough. "You can just get me to chemo. I'm sick of waiting today," I told her. Her helpful response was, "Well, you can go. You don't have to wait for Dr. Griggs." I looked at my husband, and then I looked at her, and out came, "Well, I didn't wait an hour in the waiting room to see *you*." The nurse quickly exited the room, and my doctor promptly entered, saying, "We've been wondering when you would get upset." At the time, I didn't understand why they'd expected me to be angry. But looking back, I see that it's necessary to process the unfairness of it all.

I had my husband take a picture of me in the examination room after the oncologist left. The next week, I took it to my life-portrait class. I scooted all the way to the back of the room and started frantically drawing. The instructor noticed and said, "I know you're not drawing the model that's here today." I said, "Nope, I'm not." He replied, "Well, can I see it?" It was right around my birthday—which is also World Cancer Day, February 4th. In the drawing I had tried to show my anger in a comical way: as steam coming out of my ears, spiraling and rising past my furrowed brow. He kind of chuckled and gave me a few tips to soften it.

Even the nicest people who go through this need to release their anger at some point. I had to wait until my psyche and body were ready to deal with the complexities of my layered story.

So that's what the first picture was. After that, I added more pictures that reflected the emotional parts of my healing. I tend to have a heavy hand working in charcoal, so a lot of the pictures are very dark; but in many ways it was a dark season for me, emotionally and physically.

In one drawing, I'm sitting in a chemo chair. They're nice, comfy chairs—heated blankets were my favorite—but you're surrounded with IV poles, and every time a bag gets down to a certain level, there's beeping. I would often be sitting next to people who would have lots of visitors, and they would be yapping away; so I drew a picture of me sitting in the chair, and the whole background is filled with type font: *Beep, beep, yap, yap, beep, beep, yap, yap.*

There's another one I drew, with me behind an examination-room curtain, that's about having my lymph nodes removed. I found the medical posters at the hospital fascinating, especially the ones about the lymphatic system, which I didn't know much about. In addition to chemo and radiation, I did six months of lymphedema therapy, which I needed because I had 29 lymph nodes removed under my left armpit. In the picture, half of me is behind a curtain that acts as an X-ray, with the outline of my arm raised—showing all the lymph nodes, or lack of, in that area.

I've been a swimmer for as long as I can remember. I feel at home in the water. So after I healed from surgery, I returned to the pool, pausing only during radiation. Regular workouts have played a crucial role in my healing, mentally and physically. They have also been the best therapy for my lymphedema. At first I always wore a swim cap, as I'd done when I had hair. But one day, I went to the pool in the middle of the day and it was all older gentlemen there. Most of them were balding or bald, and I just thought, *This is ridiculous. Why am I covering my head with this hot cap? They're swimming bald, and they have no shame. Why should I?* So I took it off. I remember this one man encouraging me, in a thick foreign accent: "You are so beautiful." It was empowering for me at the time to embrace what my body was going through and be more accepting of it. I also remember a lady in the locker room asking, "Are you a speed racer or something?" and pointing to my bald head. I don't know any females that shave their heads to swim faster, but I chuckled and decided people could think what they wanted.

The summer after my main treatment, we moved to Colorado. We loved living with my sister, but it was never meant to be long-term. We had always dreamed of moving out west, so we both applied to jobs. As it turned out, I was picked up for teaching right away, and we figured my husband's employment would not be far behind. We packed up all our things and headed west for a new start. I taught the whole year while he was at home applying for jobs, a process that took longer than we expected. I would go to work and teach, then go to the hospital and get my Herceptin infusion, and come home. He did all the cooking, cleaning, and running kids around. He did everything for that year. Looking back, I think if he had gotten a job first and I had waited longer, I probably wouldn't have pushed myself so hard to get back into normal life. I don't know if I could've done it without him being so supportive. My last week of teaching, he was hired for a great job. I finished school on a Friday, and he started the next Monday—the first day of my summer vacation. The timing was amazing.

There's been so much change in my life. Even though I was longing for something new and different, I had a lot of joy in that community in Michigan. Whenever you make major transition in your life, medical or physical, moving or a new job, you have to learn what defines you—what makes you, *you*. I've realized that the things that bring me joy and give me life are being with my family, being in a faith-based community, making art—not just teaching it but making it for myself—and being in the pool. Those things are things that are true to my core, and so I learned that I have to find a way to make them happen, wherever I am and in whatever state I'm living.

People made a big deal about the cancer. When they heard that word and saw the diagnosis, I think that they assumed it was the hardest thing that I was going through at the time, but it really wasn't. I feel like it gave me the space that I needed to transition, leaving the community I was in and entering a new space. There were deeper things going on in my relationships, my spiritual life, and our vocations that were much harder to process and overcome. During that season, I felt like I had a lot of support and a lot of people around me saying "How can I help?"—because they understood or could imagine how hard cancer would be. But it was really many things together that made the season hard. When you're diagnosed, a team of doctors and professionals comes together to review your case and recommend the best treatment plan; all you really have to do is show up and live through the treatment plan. But the other things in life are much muddier. You're on your own to figure out those decisions.

Once treatment was over, a lot of that support went away, even though I was still struggling with other things and learning how to move on from this life-changing and full-stop experience.

I was pretty firm in my Christian faith before I was diagnosed with cancer. Do I still believe in a higher God? Yes. Do I still believe in Jesus? Do I still believe he has a plan for me? Yes. Do I see where it's going? No, I have no idea. I feel like I'm still walking forward, but my steps are weaker and slower. When I remember the events on that paper wreath, they remind me that an all-knowing God is weaving the leaves of my story together. I have no doubt that at some point I'm going to understand, on a deeper level, why this is my story. I've come through it feeling like I know who I am. I have a firm understanding of what I believe. I don't need to paint a perfect picture, saying my life is great and everything's rosy and it's going to be always be like that—but I can say, "Hey, there's joy in the struggle, too. There's faithfulness in the hard times."

When Poetry Is Surgery With a Pen

Name: Barbara Bowen

Town: San Antonio, Texas

Diagnosis: Breast cancer; stage 3, ER+, PR+, Her2+ ("triple positive")

Age at diagnosis: 40

Age now: 42

I am a poet. Because I'm not paid for this, people like to call it a hobby. I hesitate to define it that way—very few poets are paid to write. I would actually consider myself a poet before I'd consider myself a trade-show manager, which is what I do professionally. I've been writing poetry since about 8th grade, but I wasn't much good until later. Initially it was a way to spew emotions onto the page. I was an awkward kid and needed a safe space for expression. Then I had a brilliant teacher in my junior year of high school, Carol Mengden, and she showed me how to take that spew and turn it into craft.

BEST ADVICE: Information is overrated. It was probably better that I didn't really know what I was getting into with chemo.

In 2016, a friend and I started a project for National Poetry Month called This City Is a Poem. We share daily writing prompts on Facebook and invite certain poets to respond in advance, so we can post their work. It helps encourage people to write poetry daily, and it helps make poetry accessible to people who maybe don't go to the library or can't afford books.

That same year, I turned 40. I took an amazing birthday trip to Alaska. It was beautiful and cold, and I felt great. Two days after I got back, I had my first official, "Hooray, you turned 40—let's squash your boobs" mammogram, and the result was that they found something suspicious in my right breast, so I had to go back for a second mammo.

I was pretty zen between scans, but after the second mammo, I was a little anxious. I told some core friends, "Would you please keep me in your thoughts? This is probably because I drink a lot of tea, but you never know." Then the doctor said she had to do a biopsy. That happened two days after Christmas. They offered to get me in sooner, but I didn't want to ruin the holidays for myself.

I got my diagnosis on December 30th, 2016. I wasn't surprised that it was positive. The first doctor said, "Oh, it's really tiny. You'll probably just get a lumpectomy and radiation."

Then they sent me in for more testing and told me it had spread to my lymph nodes. I would need a PET scan, to make sure that it wasn't anywhere else.

The progression didn't surprise me. I couldn't really tell you why it didn't. I think I was dissociating. I would constantly talk about myself without really thinking about it as me. I'd get a little jolt when I remembered it was. I still do this, actually. I think it's just a way of coping. Like there's this terrible thing, and it must be a super-close friend of mine going through it—oh no, wait, that's *me* we're talking about. I think that's part of how I got through it.

January was a bunch of tests and consults and all that business. At that point, the worst part was just waiting to have a plan. A friend who'd gone through breast cancer said, "Here's a couple of websites that were good resources. Here's a support group to join." By then, I was starting to freak out. Eventually I joined that support group, but at first I was too overwhelmed. I looked up breastcancer.org, I think, for basic definitions and treatment info. I opened up a page that was all about "What is chemo, and how does it work?" I took a quick look, said, "This is scary as hell," and closed that window.

Of course, what do you know—I started chemo in early February, and I still have the port in. It still hurts and twinges. Ultimately, I had six rounds of TCHP chemo, a unilateral mastectomy, radiation, and then a DIEP-flap reconstruction surgery with revisions—while getting Herceptin throughout.

I chose unilateral surgery because there was nothing cancerous present in the left breast. I talked to my oncologist, Amy Lang, a goddess in breast cancer treatment. I was like, "OK, tell me one more time there's no reason to take off the left breast because I'm not likely to develop cancer there." She said, "No, you are unlikely to develop breast cancer in the left breast. If you're going to get cancer again, it's probably going to be somewhere else." Statistically, if it's going to happen, it's going to happen somewhere that branched off the lymph system.

I chose DIEP-flap reconstruction after a plastic surgeon told me that a third of all implants fail if they follow radiation. This surgeon specialized in DIEP flaps, and they had a 99% success rate with it. I didn't want to be back in 10 years getting implants redone, and I liked the idea of using my own tissue. Keeping my nipple wasn't an option anyway. The tumor ended up being around three centimeters, and it was too close to the nipple for me to be able to keep it.

Through it all, poetry became my way to excise the cancer, to get all the pain and burden out of my head—surgery with a pen. I started after my first chemo infusion in 2017, which was really hard on me physically. I told my partner on This City Is a Poem that I was so sorry, but I wasn't going to be able to help her the way I had the previous year. She did a marvelous job keeping it up. She was the one who told me I had to write. The year prior, we had decided to make it a tradition that we'd each respond to one of the prompts ourselves. She told me to do that in treatment, and I was like, "Girl, I am doing good just to hold my head up right now." She answered, "I don't care—write something." She meant it in the best way!

So I sat in bed, looking out my window, and wrote something that responded to one of our prompts—and it ended up being about cancer. It was the first poem I wrote while in treatment. A couple of months later, I wrote another one. I gradually started building up this body of work, because I found after a while that I couldn't write about anything else. That's what's in my head right now, informing my thoughts. It's pervasive. I was initially frustrated, but I decided after a while, screw it—I'm just going to keep writing them.

Poems work in imagery. If I didn't write it out and create these visual spaces around it, then I would have all of this mess inside of me, this anger and despair and hurt. I would just be holding onto it, and I don't think that's healthy. Being able to write it out and make something that is ultimately beautiful out of something that's caused so much pain is therapeutic.

It's also helpful to me to think that all this garbage I've been through can now let me help someone else. I hope to publish a collection, eventually. I'm hoping my poems can help other patients feel understood in what they're going through.

Before treatment and since, my top passions have been writing, travel, and photography. One of the most upsetting things about my year of treatment was that I had to cancel all my travel. It angered me because I couldn't make any decisions in advance. I never knew when I might be feeling like crap. The oncologist said, "Oh, in your third week after treatment, you're going to feel pretty good, so you'll be able to take weekend trips," and that ended up completely untrue for me. It made me angry that I had to change my life for this stupid cancer.

This year, I'm still basically in active treatment because I'm taking Nerlynx. It's a new medication for HER2 positive patients that you take after Herceptin—six pills a day. Still, I have decided that this is the year of yes. If someone invites me to go visit them and I have the vacation time, I'm going. A friend of mine was getting married in Kentucky. I went. In July, another friend is getting married in New York. I'm going to that. Another friend is getting married in October in California, and I'm going to that too. It's the year of saying yes to the things that I couldn't do the year previous. Even the idea of having tickets purchased is a happy thing for me.

The poem I'm sharing with you here, **How to Go to Vegas When Vegas Is Not Where You Want to Go**, was part of the year of *yes*. It was a business trip—actually my first trip after treatment. I was irritated that my first trip was going to be Vegas. I know a lot of people love the place; it's not my favorite. But my husband loves it, and he went with me, and you know what? It was fine.

How to Go to Vegas When Vegas Is Not Where You Want to Go

Stay out late the night before.
Your friends will be charming and hilarious
and you will miss your 9:30 p.m. cutoff.
You haven't packed.
That open suitcase will lie at the back
of your mind, a gaping black maw
waiting for your t-shirts, no,
your dress shirts, no, your winter coat,
an embarrassing bright blue
that has somehow disappeared in the house.

That is what happens
when you come home from turning forty in Alaska
and the doctor calls,
asking you to come to her office.

You will get cancer, and you will lose
your coat.

Forget your coat. You have sweaters.
You can layer sweater over sweater
and anyway, it's Vegas, right?
Accuweather says it may freeze,
but what does a weather app know
about casinos rising from a desert floor,
Gamera and Mechagodzilla eyeing each other
as they leech power from settling dust?

Pack your sweater. Pack three.
Maybe one more for the flight.
Sweaters are critical. Your coat is AWOL

and you are not sure if that year
of treatment, the year you lost,
was enough to carry you past forty-five.

You lost your coat, you lost your nice leather wallet,
your short-term memory, at least
three trips—because everything is a triptych:
your sweaters, your flights out of Dodge. Everything
but those losses, which mounted up
like high scores on a video game.
With every loss, you win!
So pack six sweaters and carry three more.

Remember that when you are in Vegas,
you are still in Dodge. The constant jangling
of slot machines and press of drunk and high bodies
is not the escape you had envisioned.

When you have only eleven hours before your flight,
give up.
You will need three more pairs of underwear,
and you will remember that both your morning
and night pill boxes are empty,
but this is precisely
when you should go to sleep.

Wake up before the pet sitter arrives
so you have time to fix your new cowlick
and adjust your clothes to hide
all four body-crossing scars.

Instruct her on which cat eats the soft food
and which one is angry enough to bite.
Forget to tell her to switch off the night light

so the house can sleep at night.
Forget to tell her the dog loves her
more than he loves you.

Put on three sweaters.
Be sure one is a hoodie.
You will want to hide underneath it.

Be sure to plug in your phone
and whisper goodbye as it reboots
and reboots and dies.
Be sure you did not print any reservations
or confirmation numbers.

You may swear here.
You may blister the top of your bureau.

Check to see if you have a spouse
who can look up error codes
and book you an appointment at the Genius Bar in Vegas
while you set the bedroom on fire.

Double-check that your driver's license
is in your bag.
Make sure your insurance card is next to it,
just in case.

Double-check your phone, requiescat in pacem,
is next to those.

Now you should head to the airport,
but don't worry:
Your flight will be delayed twice. You will have time
to miss your phone.

Once you are seated on the plane,
make friends with the man next to you.
You will need his napkins
when you spill your Coke
across your book.

Your spouse will buy
you a tiny bottle of Jack.
Accept it with gratitude
and try not to spill it too.

Try not to think of your last labs
that showed persistently low blood-cell counts.
Try not to think of stale casino air.
Pull up your hoodie.

Think of forests, rain, fog,
an ocean opening up before you.

I Had No Health Advocate,
So Now I Help Others

Name: Gabriela Perez-Espinosa

Town: Moreno Valley, California

Diagnoses: Non-Hodgkin's lymphoma; Hodgkin's lymphoma

Age at diagnosis: 26, then 30

Age now: 35

I was 25. I had been with my boyfriend for about five years, and we had just had our first child. My son was about two or three months old when I started feeling sick. I had developed a persistent cough, and my boyfriend's mother kept insisting I go to the doctor. I thought, *OK, now I have a child—I have to take care of myself.*

My doctor treated me for a common cold, but after some time with no improvement, I went back and had an X-ray done. Something was visible on the X-ray, so I also had a CT scan. I remember so clearly the day the doctor called me with the results. I was working mornings at the time; my boyfriend and I rotated our work shifts so we could both care for our son. I had just gotten home, and my son was sleeping. My boyfriend ran upstairs to take a shower and get ready for his day.

That's when the call came. My doctor had

BEST ADVICE: Don't get lost in the depressing statistics and stories. Fight for your own ending.

seen something very suspicious in my lungs. She said, "This could be a very serious infection, or it could be cancer." She referred me to a lung specialist. I hung up from that conversation and stared for a long moment into my son's sleeping face. I just couldn't believe it. Then I ran upstairs to my boyfriend, pulled open the shower curtain, and started crying. He immediately panicked: "What happened? Where's the baby?" I just leaned into him. I was too shocked to speak. I still get emotional thinking about that day. It feels like the moment my life turned upside down.

A few days later, I met with the lung specialist. The first thing he asked was, "Are you a smoker?" When I said no, he said, "OK, then it's not cancer. You're too young for cancer." His words gave me a sense of relief. For the next several months, he treated me for pneumonia, with strong antibiotics. But my symptoms weren't going away, and my health was declining. I was having side effects from the medication, was severely anemic, and was constantly fatigued. Psychologically, I was in a bad place as well. Thankfully I sought counseling for my depression and anxiety. I hated being sick and not having answers. I'm so grateful that I had a supportive partner. He played both dad and mom role for our son and allowed me to focus on me.

After several more months, the lung specialist said, "Well, you're not getting better. The only other treatment option would be to remove the upper-left lobe of your lung." Being naïve, and just desperately wanting to feel better, I said, "OK, let's do it. Whatever it takes. I just want to feel normal again."

A few days before surgery, I had a bad dream. I was going in for surgery, and they opened me up, and the doctors said, "She's full of cancer" and closed me back. I talked to my boyfriend about the dream and how worried and scared I was. He told me things would be OK. Then I said, "Well, if there's anything on my bucket list, it's being married. If things go wrong, just marry me before you pull the plug."

We had talked about marriage before but hadn't been ready financially, and then there was the baby to focus on. At that moment he said, "Well, if you want to get married, we can go to the courthouse." I thought he was joking, but he was serious. He reminded me that I was the one who had always wanted to wait until we could have a big wedding. I told him I was joking and would rather wait. But two days before my surgery, I said, "You know what? Let's go to the courthouse." We got married the day before my surgery, in jeans, with just enough people to sign as our witnesses.

I have a vague memory of waking up after surgery. I was in a patient room and saw my mom in the corner. She watched over me and noticed I was struggling to breathe as time went on. She questioned the nurse on several occasions about whether that was normal and if I was OK, but the nurse seemed to brush her off. Finally, after an hour or two, my mom got desperate and started roaming the hospital, trying to find someone who spoke Spanish and would listen to her. She found someone, a doctor, and dragged her to my room. With one look at me from the doorway, the doctor called a code blue. By that point, I wasn't getting enough oxygen, and they were rushing to intubate me. I could hear my mom screaming, "Gaby, Gaby!" but I had no clue what was going on. I was panicking as I struggled to breathe. I tried opening my eyes but just saw dark silhouettes. There was so much commotion with the doctors and nurses, but I was drawn to my mom's voice. She kept saying, "Think of your baby. Think of your baby." I was terrified. I didn't want to leave him.

My next memory is of waking up with my wrist tied to the bed, tubes down my throat, and IV lines everywhere. I looked around and saw my husband standing next to me, just watching my monitors. The look on his face still haunts me. He looked so worried, so sad, so hurt. I shrugged my shoulders to catch his attention. "You want to know what happened?" he said. I nodded, or at least tried to. "You weren't breathing," he said. Then I just closed my eyes. I believe that's the moment I began to go numb. I had no real understanding of what was going on, but by the look on his face and the condition I was in, I knew it wasn't good.

The first few days I was in ICU were rough. My declining health lead the doctors to believe I had stage 4 lung cancer and that I was not going to make it. They told my family my diagnosis and advised them to start making my funeral arrangements. But on the fourth day, once they received the biopsy results from the tumor, the doctors switched the diagnosis and prognosis. As relieved as my family was to find out that my condition was not terminal, it was hard for them to understand how the doctors could have been so wrong and yet so confident.

Meanwhile, I was in and out of sedation and unaware of the emotional turmoil my family had just been through. I started getting weaned off the medication around day six. I recall bits and pieces of my eight days in the ICU. It all blended into one big nightmare, with me too confused, scared, and numb to really comprehend what was going on. I remember a nurse asking me if I would "be good" if she removed the restraints from my wrists. I remember being extubated. I remember walking around the hallways because the doctor said I had to walk to be able to leave. I also remember my brother and my husband giving me the news of what I had. I remember thinking, *What is lymphoma?* Honestly, I wasn't even aware we had lymph nodes. I looked at my husband and said, "What stage?" And he said, "Stage 4," and I remember thinking, *Well, that's not good.*

My husband told me treatment would start two weeks after I was released from the hospital, to allow my body to heal from the surgery. I had no reaction to the news. I was still on autopilot—too numb to think or feel anything, just doing what I had to do to get home and better for my son.

I soon met with my oncologist. Talk about bedside manner. The first thing he said was, "So, you just had surgery. Had we known it was cancer, we wouldn't have removed your lung. We would have treated you with chemo." To hear that my surgery had been completely unnecessary was extremely traumatic. But I couldn't let the anger sink in. I think my husband was angry enough for both of us. He took it very hard. Everyone would tell me how well I was handing it, but I honestly wasn't handling it at all. I was just going through the motions.

My treatment plan consisted of eight rounds of a drug cocktail called R-CHOP. The day I went for my first treatment, I met with my oncologist for about 45 minutes; then he took me over to the "chemo suite." As we walked, he said, "You're sure you want to go through with this? You know there's a high chance you'll be sterile afterward, right?" I stopped walking and said, "What?" I was shocked. It was the first time he had ever said this.

"An option would be to freeze your eggs," he said, but he warned me it would delay my treatment. I felt confused and at a loss for words. Thankfully my sister-in-law jumped in, saying, "Can she have a few minutes to think about this?" They gave me 10 minutes in the waiting room to decide. So, there I was, with my mother, sister-in-law, and husband. I looked at my husband, who said, "It's up to you, babe. Whatever you feel is right, I'll support you."

Then I looked at my mom, who said, "You have your baby already. Just be thankful. He's such a blessing. Get yourself better." Then I look at my sister-in-law, who said, "You're so young. You're probably going to want more kids." I was pressured to decide my future, and the future of my little family, in just a few minutes. I felt awful.

I pushed aside my emotions and tried to focus on the fact that I had to get better. I moved forward with chemo that day as planned, praying that somehow, I'd come out of it still able to have children. I walked into the chemo suite—and it all hit me. There was no privacy. All the patients were elderly. I just felt I didn't belong there. I ran to the bathroom to cry and was just saying to myself that I couldn't do it, I didn't want to do it. Yet I knew it wasn't the time to throw myself a pity party. I went to the sink, washed my face, looked in the mirror and said out loud, "You have to do this."

I did four rounds of treatment and then had a PET scan. My oncologist called me two days later and said, "You need to come in." I was scared. But when I went in, he said, "I just wanted to tell you the good news in person. You're in remission." I cried happy tears. But then I was immediately like, "OK, now what?" He told me I'd have a CT scan and do labs every three months. Those scans became my security blanket. I would have had one every day if I could have, just to have the peace of mind and know that I was still OK. Eventually he shifted them to every six months so that I wouldn't get too much radiation exposure.

My experience with the lung specialist had made me realize how important it was for me to advocate for myself, instead of trusting doctors blindly. When I spoke up with my oncologist about something that concerned me, he didn't react well. He told me, "You need to believe what I say. If I tell you today the sky is green, you should believe it's green. If I tell you it's brown, you go with brown." And I said, "No, we're not doing that—because I believed it was pneumonia for how long, and look what happened."

So I got a new oncologist. She understood my anxiety and always answered all my questions. When I worried about a relapse, she would reassure me that I was fine. We continued with my routine of blood work, CT scans, and follow-ups.

Two and a half years after my diagnosis, I found out I was pregnant. As excited as I was, it was also a scary time. I could no longer have CT scans, so I was left to settle for blood tests. The pregnancy went smoothly, and our family was blessed with a baby girl. She completed our family unit, and I felt like I was given a second chance to be the "good mom" I so desperately wanted to be.

A few months later I had a CT scan—and then a few weeks later, I had an appointment with my oncologist. She was reviewing my scan and noticed something around my chest. She said, "I'm sure it's nothing, but I know you and your anxiety. We'll do a PET scan just to be safe." The PET scan showed active cancer in my neck and chest. It was like horrible deja vu. My son was 11 months old when I was first diagnosed, and now my daughter was 11 months old. I have to say, as a parent, one of the scariest feelings is not knowing if you will be around for your child's first birthday. I had to experience that fear twice.

Right off the bat, the doctor's take was that the non-Hodgkin's had come back, and she started planning treatment for that. She warned that I was looking at a stem cell transplant, radiation, and very harsh chemo. But they did a biopsy on the lymph nodes in my neck before taking the next step. Surprisingly, it showed that it wasn't a relapse. This time it was Hodgkin's. (Hodgkin's and non-Hodgkin's are different types of lymphomas.)

It's very rare to be diagnosed with both of these, and it made my treatment plan very difficult. Some of the medication that I had already received with my first chemo treatment conflicted with the ideal ABVD cocktail that I needed for the Hodgkin's. My doctor tried doing research and couldn't find another case like mine.

She referred me to City of Hope in L.A. for a second opinion. I met with their team, and they told me if I did a stem cell transplant, I'd be in the hospital for three months getting the strongest chemo possible; then they'd give me the transplant and hope that it saved me. "What are the chances of me surviving that?" I asked. They said, "Fifty percent." I didn't like those odds. Instead, we opted to do just half the recommended amount of the Hodgkin's cocktail and radiation from my neck to chest.

Treatment lasted about four months; thankfully, I was told once again that I was in remission. But at one of my first follow-ups after treatment ended, my doctor threw me another curveball. She told me that City of Hope had written her a letter. "They believe you were misdiagnosed originally," she said. Their theory was that I didn't have non-Hodgkin's the first time around but a third kind of lymphoma, Gray Zone, which is an extremely rare combination of both Hodgkin's and non-Hodgkin's. "What does this mean?" I asked. And she said, "Nothing really, because we probably would have treated the non-Hodgkin's first, since it is the most aggressive."

It's been difficult for me to process that information. If I accept that theory, it means I was never actually in remission the first time. The first treatment cleared the non-Hodgkin's cells, but the Hodgkin's ones were still there. It's painful for me to think of all the times I was reassured that I was fine when I wasn't. My journey between the two diagnoses could have been very different; I would have been more on guard. I might have sought a second opinion. But again I cannot let the negativity and hurt consume me. Maybe it could have been worse. If the initial treatment had been more aggressive, it might have left me sterile, or I might have had more side effects; there are endless "what ifs." I was left with my scars, my fears, my anxiety, and a little lung; but I choose to focus on the fact that I have two healthy and beautiful kids and have been allowed more time with them.

Although rough, my journey has been a learning experience. I have been going to school online since I was pregnant with my son. During treatment, I was struggling and was practically failing my classes. My school counselor advised me to push forward and said, "Your employer's not going to care what grades you got. They're just going to care that you got the degree." So I kept going, but I ended my bachelor's program with a low GPA.

When I finished treatment, I decided I wanted to pursue a career as a medical-oncology social worker. I want to be the advocate voice that I had lacked during my journey. But it turned out I needed a 3.0 GPA to get into the program. I had the option of redoing my bachelor's or doing another master's first. I completed a master's in human services, increased my GPA, and am now working on my second master's. Honestly, though, it was a very expensive and time-consuming detour. Looking back, I wish I had taken time off from school during treatment, so I didn't have to waste two years and who knows how many thousands of dollars. I plan to graduate in 2021.

There's another happy ending to mention. In 2017, my husband and I finally had the wedding I'd always wanted—in a church, with a big outdoor reception afterward, surrounded by many of our family and friends.

Medicine Men & the Cultural Barriers to Good Care

. . . .

Name: Ardith Tom

Town: Gallup, New Mexico

Diagnosis: Endometrial cancer

Age at diagnosis: 25

Age now: 34

I'm Native American, from the Navajo Nation. I was born and raised on the Indian reservation in New Mexico. Cultural preservation was important to my parents. My mother and father are Navajo. Their grandparents suffered from cultural assimilation. Growing up, we were told stories about our grandparents as Navajo children torn from their families and forced into boarding schools. The children were forced to abandon their Native American identities and cultures. They were not allowed to speak their language or practice rituals. The stories stressed the importance of ensuring the survival of my culture. My siblings and I were taught, and practice, traditional customs. This became challenging when I was diagnosed with cancer.

WORST ADVICE: "Just feel grateful because you're alive." Like I shouldn't have a bad day. Like if you have negative thoughts, or you're feeling some type of way about something, you should just be happy—because, well, you survived. What? No. If one day I wanna feel like crap, guess what? I'm gonna feel like crap. But the next day I will get up and I will move forward.

I had just moved home to Gallup, New Mexico, from college, and was working as a hotel general manager. I wanted to get settled into a relationship, start a family, and move into that phase in my life. And then the diagnosis came.

The symptoms had started when I was in college. At 20, I stopped having a menstrual cycle. I kept having pap smears, which were coming back irregular—but not enough to signify cancer. Since endometrial cancer is uncommon for someone my age, doctors considered everything else first. I was just learning about being an adult. I had never had sex, and they were asking me all kinds of invasive personal questions I wasn't prepared for: "Are you pregnant? Have you had an abortion? What's your sexual history?" It took my innocence away. To learn about your body in that way is traumatizing. They didn't seem to believe me when I told them I wasn't sexually active.

This continued for about four years, and I guess in all that time, the tumor inside of my uterus was growing. Finally, one day I started bleeding uncontrollably, and I drove 25 miles to the closest ER. It was a very small, rural hospital, so they had to transfer me to another one. There, they decided to do a biopsy inside my uterus. That's when they found it: a tumor the size of a cantaloupe. I couldn't feel it inside me at all.

After so many years of not knowing what was wrong with me, I actually felt a sense of relief to hear that I had cancer: *Oh my goodness, yay! I'm not crazy after all, and there's finally an answer to what we need to do.* Then I told my mom and my sister, and both of them just fell apart. And it made me laugh, because I was like, "That should be me, but OK. I'll be fine. Don't worry."

I called the doctor, and she told me I had to have a hysterectomy. "You are really young. Have you thought about having a family?" she asked. I had always envisioned myself being a mom. I love taking care of people and had thought about what to name my child for as long as I could remember. "So what do you want to do?" she asked.

She explained that I could freeze my eggs, but waiting was risky since the tumor was growing fast. She also told me it was possible that the cancer might be in my eggs. That sealed the deal: "If there's a chance my child could have cancer, then no."

I sat there for a minute, realizing that my whole life had just changed—everything I thought I knew I was going to do, everything I thought I was going to get to be. I didn't even have time to wrap my head around it. All of a sudden, the surgery was scheduled for two weeks out, and I was putting in my leave at work.

Where I grew up, health care is hard to access. It's geographical. You have to drive for hours to Albuquerque. People who have cancer tend to end up waiting until it's in its advanced stages. So when people hear "cancer," they automatically assume you're going to die. Before I had surgery, my grandma brought a medicine man to her home to see me. She believes in the ancient traditional healings. My grandma told the medicine man, "She has cancer." He said, "All right, I'll take it out." And I was like, "You're gonna take it out? *What?*" My grandma said, "Just trust him. He'll take it out."

"Do I have a choice in this?" I asked her. "No," she answered.

He brought out his tools—Indian arrowheads, crystals, smoke pipes. My mind was full of conflicting thoughts. *Am I wrong to run out of here saying I don't believe this? Do I believe it? I don't know. I don't have a choice. Do I have a choice? Am I gonna upset my family?* I wondered if maybe I should do it just to give my family comfort, because there were so scared for me. Then he brought out a large stone arrowhead and pointed it at me.

I had seen some of these ceremonies before. The medicine man doesn't cut the cancer out but makes a ceremonial cut, so that the Indian medicine can enter and heal you. For breast cancer, they use hot ash to "burn out the tumors." These people do it, and they believe in it. They were raised on this faith, and it's hard to know if you should question it.

"I'm gonna cut it out of your stomach," he said. "It going to hurt, but you need to sit still. We're going to carve it out of you."

This was too much. I stood up and said, "No, I cannot do this. Thank you, Grandma. I don't know what you paid this man. I don't mean to disrespect you or disrespect what you believe—what we believe, our culture. But I don't believe this. I don't. I can't."

My family and the medicine man were staring at me, as though by standing down I was asking to die. My mom started crying. But I couldn't do it. I walked outside. My dad came out after me. He is a very reserved man and doesn't say much. But he said, "You know what? I would've pulled you out of there too. You are not going to do this." And he hugged me. It was exactly what I needed to feel I had done the right thing.

I believe in my creator. I believe in the Holy people. And I believe in Mother Earth. But I noticed that the practices of this medicine man weren't even part of the traditions we were raised on. Navajo healers prayer through singing and chanting. This healer wanted to cut a part of my stomach open.

My mom reached out to a friend, and they found a gentleman who lived about an hour and half from our house. He invited us to his hogan, a traditional Navajo home made of wood and mud, with a dirt floor and a wood stove in the middle. We prayed there, and it was beautiful. We smoked cedar and sweet tobacco. And we sang, he sang, all night long. He prayed for my healing. "Bless her with the strength to get through this. Let the surgery go well. Let the surgeon have a great day. Let the surgeon wake up early and feel good about himself, so he goes in focused," he said, along with other things like that. It was empowering. I looked at him and said, "Thank you. I can leave here knowing that I'll be OK." I was so grateful for that time with my family.

The surgery did go great, but things got much worse afterward. The doctor said she wanted me to have a type of radiation called vaginal brachytherapy as a precaution. "You'll go through five cycles, and you'll have only a .1% chance of it ever coming back," she said. I thought, *We went this far—let's do it.* Unfortunately, I had no idea what I was walking into and what it would take away from me.

In brachytherapy, they insert a probe into your vagina. It's super painful and takes away any sense of privacy, especially for someone who has never been sexually active. I didn't know what having a probe inserted there would be like or what it would do to that part of my body. It's radiation inside your most private part. The initial radiation therapy is only about 15 minutes, but the prep is two hours. You have doctors, nurses, and techs in and out while you lay still on that bed with that probe inside you, with Velcro straps holding it in place. You're covered, but it's still so embarrassing and invasive. You can't move. If you move, there's the chance of it shooting radiation to other parts of your body—potentially damaging your rectum, damaging your bladder, and on like that. I did this five times over the course of a month.

When I was done, I wanted to forget the last six months had ever happened. I quit my job and started traveling with my sister, Cheri. We were traveling, writing, doing things that we've wanted to do. We moved to Albuquerque. We got new jobs. I totally blocked out being sick and never told new people what had happened. It finally felt like I was in control again and the cancer was just a hiccup. That part was done. But nothing could have prepared me for what happened next.

I had been in remission for about 10 months. My sister and I were living well and having adventures. One day, we were going to a wine festival and I just got sick. I felt like I was going to faint. I went home and started having terrible pain in my stomach. When I got a fever, I went to the ER. Going over my medical history, I told them, "A year ago I had cancer, but it's gone."

Their tests weren't finding anything, so finally they said, "As a precaution, let's do a CT scan." When the doctor came back with results, he said, "Ardith, you have a tumor growing inside of you. And the reason you have such a bad fever is the tumor is infected." He told me they didn't know much but that it looked like a mini basketball. Back to the cantaloupe again; I guess it likes that shape. My oncologist came to the hospital the next day and said, "I'm not going to lie to you, we don't know what's going to happen next. But it's there—it's back and growing fast." She told me I'd do chemo right away, plus radiation. The diagnosis now was metastatic endometrial cancer. I was about to turn 27.

I've had long hair my entire life. In Navajo tradition, hair is a symbol: You're given long, beautiful straight hair because you want a long, straight life. Hair is sacred, so I had never had a haircut or had it dyed. You might think I'd be freaked out even more than most people about losing my hair. But actually, I was really excited. I was like, "I can have the most awesome haircut ever." I hated the first cut I got, but then got it fixed—at Walmart of all places. I was so proud of my hair. I walked out of there glowing.

The first round of treatment lasted a month. During that time, my sister got a cold, so she went back to Gallup in order not to infect me. After a week, she had gotten worse instead of better. She went to the clinic, and they told her she had mumps. Then she had an inflamed lymph node in her neck, and they told her it was bronchitis. The next diagnosis was mono. Finally, we were back at home together for the first time since my chemo had started. Cheri said, "Mom, my throat doesn't feel well." My mom took a look and said, "Oh, Cheri, it looks like it's narrowing. Let's go to the clinic."

The doctors at the clinic in Gallup told my family that if we hadn't brought her in, she would have suffocated in her sleep. Her lymph nodes had swollen to the size of golf balls. They flew Cheri and my mom to the nearest hospital, 140 miles away—the University of New Mexico Hospital. That's where she found out she had acute lymphoblastic leukemia.

My dad, who like I said is a rock, just broke down when he heard. This was during my second round of chemo, in November, 2013. They put Cheri in a clinical trial. She stayed for 75 days straight in the oncology ward, about 10 miles from where I was being treated.

I know I can't speak for my sister, but I think this must have been devastating to her. When we found out I couldn't have children, she said, "Don't worry Ardith—I'll have one for you. I'll carry one for you. Don't let that be the thing you worry about. I got you." She'd always been the strong one. My role as a sister changed very suddenly. "Cheri, we're gonna get through this together, both of us," I said.

Looking back, how my family handed those 75 days together bonded us forever. The hospital can break you. It's a healing place, but there's nothing in there that lights hope. The rooms are gloomy, with dark beige walls. We would feel just beaten from the chemo, because it was really strong. On hard days, if Cheri cried, I'd tell her, "Here's what we're gonna do next, where we're going to travel." And on my low days, she did the same for me. We were continuously in and out of hospitals together for about two years.

My whole family stepped in to keep life as normal as possible. They brought the entire Thanksgiving dinner into the waiting room of the hospital. They set out the full meal, and 25 of us had dinner there. Christmas, same thing. New Years Eve, my brother brought a bucket of party blowers and hats, but we told our family to go out and have fun without us. We both fell asleep—until 11:55, when I woke up. "Cheri, you have to get up, the countdown is going to begin." And she was like, "I don't feel good. I'm gonna go to the bathroom."

By this time it was 11:58. I sat there in my room, alone, thinking, *Am I going to see another new year? Is my sister?* And all of a sudden the door busted open, and my mom, dad, and brothers walked in. I said, "Did we make it?" And they said, "Yes, you did!" We were blowing horns, and we all hugged, and it was a great time. We left the hospital and went home that night.

Still, it was hard. Your whole appearance changes. You've lost your hair and your eyebrows; your body changes. I gained weight. My sister took a line of chemotherapy called Vincristine. It was really, really strong, and it has neurological effects at times. She had hallucinations and the worst of all the side effects they warn you about, times ten. I never wanted someone to pity me. So I fought hard. If I was in pain, I wouldn't show it. If I felt sick, I wouldn't show it. I would save face and hold strong. I come from a small town where everyone knows everyone. We didn't want to face all those people and have them feeling sorry for us.

We turned everything we could into an adventure. When we were in Texas for Cheri to have stem cell therapy, we would try new restaurants and go to shows. We'd drive to Austin to see the lake. We'd find things to see that we'd never seen before, ways to continue to live.

Finally we started getting better. Having been unemployed and in hospitals so long, we couldn't afford to live in Albuquerque anymore, so we had been traveling back and forth for treatment. We had no idea that there might be resources able to help us, financially or any other way. Finally one day I went to get my port flushed in Albuquerque, and they told me I could start doing it in a clinic in Gallup. I said, "What? I don't have to go 140 miles, almost 300 roundtrip, to get my port flushed?"

I skipped into the Gallup clinic the first time. And while I was waiting for my appointment, I saw a brochure that said, "Are you a young adult with cancer?" And I said, "Hey, yes, I am." The brochure was for Camp Make a Dream. And I thought, *Ardith you should apply. Apply to Camp Make a Dream.* I convinced my sister to apply, too, and they invited us both to participate. We went up there and met other young adults who had been through stuff as insane as our experiences. Some of our mates there had just finished a session at Camp Koru, and they were like, "You have to go. You have to." They told me it was a surf camp, and I said, "Oh, wow—I don't know if I can do that. I mean, look at me." I was at a really heavy weight at that point. "Oh, man, that'd be awesome, but I'm not gonna be on no surfboard. I don't think so." But I went to Koru. It pushed me out of my comfort zone. This girl got up and rode a wave.

I'm a strong person, but those camps showed me aspects of my strength I didn't know I had. I've done things I'd never thought were possible. I never thought I'd be on a zipline, or on a surfboard, or on the back of a horse. No, that's not me. Hiking mountains and climbing though waterfalls—no, not me. Now I look back and think, "All those things that were supposed to break you—look how far they've taken you."

As I mentioned, access to health care in rural New Mexico is very limited. Aside from the distance to services, there are the cultural barriers. We're raised to believe that there are things you don't talk about. You don't talk about being sick. You don't talk about mental health. My sister and I want to set up an organization that creates a space for people to talk about anything—and get resources and hope.

We saw people from the reservation in the hospital. They didn't have any visitors. They were scared. There was one lady who was there who didn't speak English; she only spoke Navajo. No one was there to talk to her. She had cancer in her stomach but couldn't understand the doctors or nurses. She just thought, "I'm here to die." She told my mom that. My mom was able to find out what was really happening and explain to her that she wasn't dying. Her cancer had been caught in the early stages.

We especially want to reach people out on the Navajo reservation, which crosses into four states. We want people to have the kinds of conversations we didn't get to have. We want people to get the help they need—and to have someone to talk to.

Growing Beyond the Trauma of Cancer

· ·

Name: Leslie Tysseling

Town: Murrieta, California

Diagnosis: Acute promyelocytic leukemia (APML, APL)

Age at diagnosis: 33

Age now: 37

I was a stay-at-home mom to a 4-year-old when I was diagnosed with leukemia in the fall of 2015. I had experienced symptoms starting in 2014, but in the spring of 2015, they got much more serious. I started having some trouble breathing; and my head felt like it was going to explode, with no relief for four months. I had night sweats and joint pain. My calf hurt, and I was lethargic. Four months before I was diagnosed properly, deep purple bruises started appearing on my body. I had been to multiple doctors, not getting anywhere. My local doctors were starting to make me feel like a hypochondriac.

Nine days prior to my diagnosis, I was in so much agony that I dragged myself to my local emergency room at 4 a.m. I told the ER doctor all my symptoms and showed him my bruises. He asked me if I was in a healthy relationship. I tried to explain that no one was beating me—I was sick! He appeared tired, somewhat robotic, and probably bored with my explanation of symptoms. He sent me away, telling me I needed to finish the antibiotic regimen I was already on. I was barely able to walk out of the ER and felt completely defeated. In addition to all my other symptoms, nine days later my collarbone hurt and was causing me agony. My husband Googled my symptoms, told me I had leukemia, and convinced me to go back to the ER.

Finally I did get diagnosed with cancer, on a Friday evening, in the exact same emergency room I had visited nine days prior. I was diagnosed

> BEST ADVICE: All our work to heal may not restore what we had before, but as long as we keep going, a beautiful, stronger, wiser, and even shinier version of our lives will show through. You are stronger than your pain; and even if you're hanging by a string, you're still fighting. That fight is worth it. It pains us, cuts us, burns, scars us—and also helps us discover hidden blessings and awakens our greatest joy. Remember to really feel: to break down, cry, fall apart—it's OK. Then wake up and show up. You can do it. More is to come. Keep adding to your story.

by a different and better doctor who ran proper tests. By that time, the leukemia was so advanced that it had caused strokes and multiple blood clots. My blood counts were so low, I was told I might have only about five days to live. I would learn that the type of cancer I had, acute promyelocytic leukemia (called APML or APL), is a subtype of acute myeloid leukemia (AML), a cancer of the white blood cells.

I was rushed by ambulance, on a transport stretcher, to Loma Linda University Hospital, in Loma Linda, California. The oncology unit was full, and I was admitted to the ER only after my husband told them, "They brought her here in an ambulance because the first hospital said she was critical enough that she needed immediate treatment. We are not going home until she sees an oncologist."

I thought I would go home that night. Instead, I didn't leave the hospital for two months. No one can fully prepare for a cancer diagnosis—but I never even got to go home to grab a toothbrush. And I didn't get to do the thing I wanted to do the most: talk to my son and attempt to explain what was happening. I wanted to tell him that I was very sick and the hospital was going to help me; to hug him one more time, cuddle with him, and tell him I love him more than anything.

I vividly remember this combination of peace and fear coming over me when I was diagnosed. I was scared but ready to fight. I also had a sense of relief, after being misdiagnosed for almost a year and in so much pain for months. Hopefully it wasn't too late. I was ready and had to be strong. I had a precious little boy who had just turned four and a husband who needed me to gear up mentally.

In the ER, it took a brave nurse breaking the rules and paging a doctor on another floor, who in turn paged an on-call doctor at his home, for me to get to see an oncologist. When the doctor who was at home pulled up my levels on his device, he was overcome with determination to come to the hospital to help me. He knew I was so close to death. He couldn't let me die.

Despite their not having an oncology room available, because I had no immune system anymore, a doctor made room. They moved me to a neutropenic hospital room—a room that has to go through a thorough sterile disinfectant protocol. I had a bone marrow biopsy, which eventually revealed the extremely rare form of cancer I have. Typically only 1,000 people in the U.S. get diagnosed with this per year.

I started chemotherapy right away. Three specialists came in on a Saturday to get me up and running. What they ordered were their best guesses, because my bone marrow results were needed for a real diagnosis; but there was no time. The action of the first ER nurse paging the doctors put into motion the steps that saved my life over the next 24 hours. I credit many medical professionals at Loma Linda for making it possible for me to begin the fight and start induction, in neutropenic hospital room 6. Thank you!

I was in that room, on the 9th floor, for two months, quarantined.

I do not recall how I got to that floor or who changed me into a gown. I remember coming to on day five or six with greasy hair and unbrushed, slimy teeth, unable to get out of bed. In the next few days, I barely got to see my son and had limited time with visitors. Blood vessels in my eyes had hemorrhaged, turning the sclera red. Initially, since I had red eyes and was surrounded by monitors, my son was scared of the hospital and of me. Being away from home and my son, plus seeing the trauma this caused him, was one of the most difficult parts of my experience. I felt guilty, and it pulled on every emotion possible.

I had blood draws daily at 4 a.m., blood and plasma transfusions, EKGs, and two chemotherapy treatments every day. MRIs and echocardiograms. Plus steroids, lots of prescriptions, and no fresh veggies or fruit or flowers, due to being neutropenic. My every move was watched and accounted for. Every morning, an oncologist would come in and evaluate me—look my body over for bruising, check my levels, determine if I needed blood transfusions or platelets, order tests. I couldn't go outside or leave the 9th floor. I couldn't feel the sunshine on my skin. I wasn't at home, sleeping in my bed. I wasn't allowed to brush my teeth or shower for 13 days—and when I could, I was still a fall risk, so even going to the bathroom or showering had to be monitored. I had to surrender everything I had known or done or been.

After two months, I was far from better. In order to leave the hospital, I needed to be stable enough that they could replace my peripherally inserted central catheter (PICC) line with a chemotherapy port—a vascular-access device that's implanted under the skin. Finally they scheduled the surgery to place the port, but the morning it was to occur, the surgeon came in for a pre-op and called it off. My numbers had fallen again.

In that moment, I felt like it was over. I was giving up. In tears, I told my husband I couldn't do this anymore. I couldn't fight any longer.

We don't know how or why, except by some divine intervention, but at that moment a transport nurse wheeled a transport hospital bed to my room and said, "I'm here for patient Leslie Tysseling. I'm from interventional radiology, taking her down to get her port."

A miracle! My doctors had been trying to get me on interventional radiology's schedule for the last ten days, with no success. Nowhere on any schedule or computer was my name or surgery scheduled with them. We felt like some higher power, angels, or God himself made this possible.

As I lay on the surgical table having my chest cut open, conversing with the doctors while overwhelmed with pain, angels were with me. They were right by my side, helping me through what took place the rest of that day. I got my chemo port and then had another scheduled chemotherapy infusion.

In the late afternoon, my doctors were divided on my status. One particular doctor felt I would improve if I got to try going home. He believed more healing would take place at home. Meanwhile, attending oncologists with superior status and experience felt I needed to remain as an inpatient. I could hear them arguing outside my hospital door.

The underdogs won, and the staff discharged me at 10:30 p.m. on Thursday. I didn't even know how to get out of the hospital, because I couldn't recall getting to the 9th floor. I had to be back in less than eight hours for outpatient chemo.

Only 30% of people make it through their quarantine induction. Doctors told me I had made it through the hardest part. However, outpatient chemo was much scarier to me. I had been a human pincushion—tested, poked, infused, prodded—yet I was afraid to start outpatient chemotherapy. I was extremely sore and swollen from port placement. The area of my chest where it was placed was black, blue, purple, and swollen. All I kept thinking was, *I've had no tour of the outpatient infusion center. No one has explained what's next—and they want to insert a needle to access a swollen, bruised port site?*

I've since realized why I was so anxious. I was leaving the secure bubble of round-the-clock care to start the task of travel to outpatient chemo, Monday to Friday, for the next seven months. A couple of months prior to all this, my uncle had died at the age of 57 from one blood clot. Despite being on blood thinners, I had immense fear of clots killing me. If they didn't kill me, there were germs at home. Going home also meant I had to learn to inject my blood-thinner shot into my stomach, twice a day.

Thank you to my parents and family, who dropped everything when I got sick to come from out of state and care for my son and me. At this point, I worried about keeping up with my active son. I didn't just have leukemia—I had no immune system. I didn't want to tell my son constantly that I couldn't do things for him. He couldn't comprehend that mommy was super-sick. I felt guilty when I had to tell him that after two months of what felt to him like abandonment, I would be going back to the hospital every day for eight hours. The look in his eyes was crushing. I would pray when I arrived home from chemotherapy that I would have just enough strength to read to him and put him to bed.

Chemo started at 7 a.m. the day after my release. It became my full-time job. I was there every weekday for seven months. When I got a little bit better in 2016, I did get some weeks off—but I was taking eight chemo pills a day no matter what.

In the beginning, I wasn't strong enough to drive myself to the hospital, so one of my parents drove me while the other took care of my son while my husband was at work. Eventually my mom had to go back home—her employer wouldn't let her have more time off. She was so worried about me. She considered quitting, but I told her, "This will be over soon, and I don't want you to end up with no job."

By that point, I was strong enough to take myself and even felt like I needed the mental break I got from driving alone. Everyone worrying about my every move and every symptom, and knowing every detail of everything, was daunting. Family had become overprotective and it was exhausting me even further.

I showed up bright and early to chemo every day in the comfiest clothes possible. My head pounded, so I didn't read or write. I'd watch TV. Sometimes I would sleep. Clothing hurt. One of my chemos made my skin burn, peel, and sometimes bleed. Another drug made my head feel like I had a migraine from the fiery depths of hell.

There was a girl in her 20s who didn't have cancer but had to have infusions for another type of blood disorder. She would walk up and down the infusion center, which was huge, with 25 stations, and talk to everybody. I thought, *I need to be more like her. I can sit here and be miserable, or I can hear other people's stories and experiences.*

I had to do labs and an EKG twice a week, but I had two hours between my tests and infusions. I started using the downtime to talk to people. I would walk the hall or hospital grounds to keep up strength and find people who wanted to chat. Sometimes I went to the children's hospital. Visiting and listening to others, I made a lot of good friends. I would tear labels for the chemo nurses. "Put me to work," I told them. "I have to sit here anyway."

In your darkest moments, try to find ways to serve. In the chaotic first days, not knowing whether I would live or die, my husband took the tedious task of changing my hospital sheets for the medical staff. He saw how overworked they were and took it upon himself—in his exhausted, worried state—to serve me and the staff. Every Saturday, he ordered pizza for the unit staff. I looked forward to Saturdays, because it meant we'd made it through another week. On a restricted neutropenic diet, I could still eat pizza, and I'd have a visit from my son. Find ways to celebrate every hard moment you get through.

I started asking the doctors and nurses to call me anytime they had a new APL patient. I knew that the patient would be in quarantine for a couple months, as I had been, without many visitors. I knew how old it could get, stuck in a hospital room, blank walls, a clock staring down at you. It can feel like an eternity. One dad I visited was around my age. He had a wife and four kids; the kids, including twins, were under the age of six and not able to visit often.

Because it's a rare cancer, there aren't that many APL patients. When I arrived, I didn't get to talk to anybody who had it. I felt like that would have been hugely helpful. I wanted to tell people like this man what I would have wanted to know: That even though it can be so bad and so scary, you can get to the other side. When people first come in, you can see the fear in their eyes. I'd say to them, "It's scary, but it's not as scary as you think. I thought a lot of scary things about cancer, and they didn't all happen to me." I'd tell them that the pain and everything you give up to heal is worth it.

Finally, after seven more months, I came to my last week of chemo treatments—but in my last week, I had an abnormal EKG. Just when I was ecstatic to be finishing treatment, my follow-up echocardiogram revealed a mass in my aortic valve. I sat in my chemo chair, crushed and scared again, wondering what this meant and how it could be happening. After a few cardiologist appointments, I was diagnosed with a benign tumor. The tumor is still present; my cardiologist monitors it to this day. As life has normalized, I often forget it's there.

The infusion center had become my world. I was at the hospital for almost a year. I was only allowed to travel from the hospital to my home. You become attached to your caretakers. When my last day came, I was bawling. My doctor had become like family. He'd had me help him pick out his girlfriend's engagement ring on the Blue Nile website during one of my appointments (he told me if I was late for infusion, not to tell the nurses it was his fault). The relationships I had were just a little bit different because I was there so much.

In some semi-twisted way, cancer makes you feel grateful to be part of it—part of the cancer community. I don't know how to describe with words what it has given me. I gave up a lot, but I gained many things: perspective, more gratitude, mental strength. I tried to let go of expectations and some things from my old life, in exchange for more days to experience so much—the highs and lows of life, and seeing my son accomplish and grow.

I finished treatment in May of 2016. That summer was kind of rough. My energy was low, and my son is pretty active. It's a harder period to figure out. During treatment, you have a plan, doctors supporting you, and family and friends to help care for your household. And then—that's finished. You're thrown back into normal life, and you're not ready for it. My hematologist always told me, "You need to be able to mourn the loss of your old life and process those feelings." But no one had much guidance about how to process my new life at home.

I do not miss being an inpatient or the daily outpatient hospital visits. But I do miss the security and the understanding.

Alone, I'm critical of myself for gaining weight and not doing or accomplishing as much. I'm mean to myself. I'm frustrated with aches, pain, and emotions that are hard to process. I'm still going to many appointments. Others may not see how much a survivor is still fighting, or comprehend the strength and determination that got me here. But I'll take it all—and thank my body every day for carrying me into the future, with its pains and celebrations.

I'm grateful my son is so active. It forced me to get out of bed and face life with all its demands. It gave me a perspective that I could gain only from him, plus the joy of being with him and seeing all his new accomplishments. By fall of 2016, though, I was struggling. I had been fighting to get the energy back to get through a 15-minute TV workout, but instead of getting better, I was feeling lower and gaining weight. Eventually I was diagnosed with an autoimmune disorder called Hashimoto's. They don't know if it's coincidental or was triggered by my treatment. I started working with an integrative-medicine doctor and will eventually see an endocrinologist—another specialist to the list! My leukemia history makes this more complicated to treat, so it takes a lot of different doctors comparing notes to figure out how to move forward. Meanwhile, they don't know if I can have a second child. Most likely I cannot.

Still, I'm grateful that it's Hashimoto's, not another cancer or a relapse. In the spring of 2018, I finally got to do what I love, gardening—after a year and a half. I grow flowers, fruits, and vegetables. When I was cleared to get my hands in the dirt again, I was so happy. I had to start the garden over. I planted a lemon tree, orange bell peppers, and celery, plus pumpkins for Halloween. I love my flowers and being able to garden and work outside. It's therapeutic for me—except for weeding!

Yesterday as I was watching my son and the neighborhood kids in our backyard playing, I felt the warmth of the sun on my face. I am blessed that my neutropenic, no-sunshine, no-showering days are over. Those horrible in-patient days got me to where I am today; and somehow, the hellish moments also gave me miracles.

In recovery, I've become a Maskcara makeup artist who works with many women, including those who have or have had cancer. I had the courage to learn and work toward a goal of starting my own make-up business. I visit patients. I'm strengthened and blessed by hearing their stories. I've had more days to be here caring for and playing with my son. I've checked things off my bucket list. I've made new friends. I've also had a few more bone marrow aspirations, biopsies, and echocardiograms. It's the good with the bad—a.k.a. *life.*

I'm now two and a half years into my "new normal." I've been sorting out the trauma, healing the frustrations and deep emotions. I feel little physical reminders: My hip and knee hurt, and I have some annoying tingling from the chemo. I have tears—sometimes from frustration, but mostly from overwhelming gratitude. I am here today! I'm capable and strong enough to tackle life.

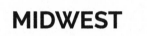

MIDWEST

Saved by a Second Opinion

Name: Gina Marie Cortese

Town: Cleveland, Ohio

Diagnosis: Giant-cell glioblastoma

Age at diagnosis: 20

Age now: 27

It was 2012, and I was home on Christmas break. I was a junior at Kent State, majoring in early childhood education. During the break I had a job at Pandora, the jewelry store. With the holiday rush, I was spending 10 to 12 hours per day on my feet. I didn't mind it. Actually, I liked it. I liked working with all the people.

One morning that month, I woke up and noticed my left toe was numb. I thought maybe I'd pinched a nerve with all those hours of standing, and I shook it off. But then I started waking up every day feeling sad and having crying jags. That was totally unlike me. I'm usually pretty happy. Also, my hair started falling out in clumps.

BEST ADVICE: I'll always remember what my neighbor Kay said to me when I was first diagnosed: "Whatever it is, you'll get through it."

I knew something was wrong, so I went to the doctor. I was 20 years old and still seeing a pediatrician. She suggested it was seasonal depression disorder. "You're probably just really stressed out from a busy schedule," she told me. "Just go back to school—you'll be fine. If things get worse, call me."

Things did get worse. I went back to school still feeling sad and not myself. The numbness spread to my other toes. Then one day, a few weeks into the new semester, I was giving a presentation to my class when I had to ask to sit down. I was lightheaded and seeing flashing lights on the floor. I tried to walk back to my desk, but my left knee gave out. I caught myself and managed to hobble to my desk.

By now I was really nervous; I knew something was seriously wrong. I limped out of the classroom and called my mom: "I don't know what to do. I'm in class and my body is giving out." She immediately called our neighbor, Kathryn—we call her Kay—who's a nurse. Kay said I should come home immediately. I called my boyfriend at the time to drive me to my parents, 45 minutes away. In the car, he rubbed my thigh to relax me, and I couldn't even feel his hand. That was the "Oh, boy, this is getting scary" moment.

From home I went straight to the ER, again taking our neighbor's advice. The doctor sent me for an MRI. The MRI tech told me I looked like I was 12, then warned me it was going to be loud. When the doctor came back with the results, she didn't tell me at first. She gathered my family outside the emergency room. I was watching through a glass window as she talked to them. They all started crying, and I panicked.

Then she came in and told me, "You have a brain mass." I immediately started crying, looking into the eyes of my family through the window. Kay had come with us. "What if I have a brain tumor? What if it's cancer, Kay?" I asked her. I remember so clearly what she answered: "Whatever it is, Gina, you'll get through it."

After that, I was transported to the main campus in an ambulance. By that time, they had gotten the brain surgeons on board. The next thing I knew, my brain surgery was scheduled for February 3rd. This was January 25th. They didn't yet know exactly what they were dealing with. From my scan, it didn't look like cancer.

The mass they removed was four centimeters, golf-ball size. Surgery was ten hours, and I remember being wheeled from surgery to the intensive care unit—and saying, "Don't go over the bumps. It's so hard." I woke up in the ICU in so much pain that I was puking all over myself. I had an unimaginable headache. They couldn't control the pain, and I was just so out of it. I couldn't read the clock or tell time. I couldn't move anything on the left side of my body. I couldn't move my arm. I couldn't move my hand.

In the midst of all this, I got the news that the mass was cancer. They would give me a month to recuperate from the surgery and do physical therapy, occupational therapy, and speech therapy. I needed to start to relearn to walk, read, and use my body. Then I'd start eight weeks of radiation, plus chemo at the same time.

I went Monday through Friday for radiation. I was on an oral chemo and an intravenous chemo for a year and a half. I had to leave school during this period and stay with my parents. At chemo, I just read magazines. But my hours at home, when I was taking the oral chemo, I filled with art. I found a lot of hobbies. I redid furniture. My mom and I would go to thrift stores and buy chairs or tables, and we would sand them down, and I would paint them. Now all my apartment furniture is pieces I've repurposed. I also took up card-making—greeting cards, birthday cards. Anything. I like to do that still. It's really fun.

I took two watercolor classes. I was always the youngest person there, alongside a bunch of old ladies and men exploring hobbies in retirement. Everybody knew I was on chemo and would ask me questions about how everything was going. I wasn't completely bald. Thanks to radiation on three-quarters of my brain, I had a mullet. The back part of my hair grew, but one side not at all, and the other I shaved because it was growing in uneven. I didn't lose my eyebrows or eyelashes, and when I wore head scarves or hats, you couldn't really tell anything was wrong.

Honestly, I took solace in being in a room full of elderly folks. I felt comfortable because I knew they understood the struggles of health. Trying to talk about being sick with people my age was awkward. People would get scared or not know what to say. But when I told older people, they were totally comforting. I never felt awkward or weird. Even now, it's hard for me to tell people I had cancer, especially guys. I haven't gone on a date where I had to tell somebody in a while, but it is very, very hard to do it. I try to mention it in passing: "Oh yeah, I'm a cancer survivor." Sometimes they ask me questions. But most of the time, people are just like, "Oh great, that's cool." And we move on. I feel like most people don't really want to know about it— and that's fine, because it's a draining story to tell.

For eight months after chemo I was stable, with a clean MRI every month. Then one month, my scan lit up. I had surgery a second time, and afterward they told me they hadn't been able to remove all the cancer. The doctors told me, "You've done the standard of care here. We don't really have any other options for you, but we can look for clinical trials." I ended up starting one at the Cleveland Clinic, which is really close to my house. I had Gamma Knife surgery, too. That's a very intense form of targeted radiation—a super-hot beam, like radiation, but 20 times stronger.

The trial was about six months—but in the middle of it, they kicked me out, because they thought they saw more cancer growing. The trial doctors wanted me to have something called NEOBLADE surgery right away. "We're gonna schedule it for next week," they told me. But my reaction was, "Oh my God, another brain surgery. No! I don't want this." I asked about the risks. A doctor said, "You could be totally paralyzed on your left side." And I said, "I'm not doing it. What happens if I don't?"

"You'll have six months to live," was his answer.

I left the office and didn't say another word the rest of the day. I just lay on the couch and cried. After that day, I didn't go back to the clinic again.

Instead, I went back to the hospital; but instead of seeing the pediatric oncologist, I went to the brain oncologist for adults. She looked at my last MRI and shook her head. "I'm not even 100% sure that it's a tumor," she said. "It could just be swelling." This was the best news I had heard in so long. My parents and I were elated.

She recommended hyperbaric oxygen therapy. You go into a chamber where you breathe in 100% oxygen. It's supposed to reduce swelling—it's similar pressure to being submerged 60 feet underwater. I had to get ear tubes put in to stop my eardrums from rupturing.

I lay in that chamber every day for eight weeks, for two and a half hours at a time. The first and second MRIs looked the same, but the third was different. It turned out that my new oncologist was right: What was showing up on the scans was swelling and leaky blood vessels, not a new mass. If I had taken the earlier recommendation of doctors who told me I had six months to live, I would have had a risky new surgery that could have paralyzed me, for no reason.

The oxygen chamber was my last treatment. That was in September of 2014. I still get MRIs every four months and visit that same oncologist. She's my lifesaver. Going to her was the best decision I ever made.

Throughout my sickness, I stayed away from online or in-person support groups. I didn't want to read about other people's experiences. I tried at first to read the cancer blog of a girl I knew growing up, but it was completely overwhelming and depressing to me. I tried a local support group, hoping to be uplifted. Instead, everybody was crying and complaining. Then one of the guys said, "My best friend's mom just died of GBM today." And I was like, "What's GBM?" "Glioblastoma," he said. I got up and walked out. That's what I had. I vowed to myself, "I am never doing anything like that, ever again."

So I didn't reach out to anybody who had cancer. I had my parents, my brother, my family, my aunts. Kay was amazing too. My boyfriend at the time was really supportive and good to me. And I had my best friends.

My attitude toward learning about my diagnosis and treatment was, "I don't want to know anything about it. I just want to do it." I never really knew what was coming at me. Gamma Knife? I had no idea. (It turned out to be the most painful experience of everything.) Brain surgery? I thought I was going to be fine. I didn't have any expectations, and that's the way I wanted it. When they were telling me all the risks and side effects of chemo, I said, "Nope, don't wanna hear it. Just tell my parents." I didn't even know what type of tumor I had. I knew if they told me, I would look it up. I didn't want to—or couldn't—process all the things that might happen. I just wanted to get it done and take things as they came.

I'm so happy I did that. If I had looked it up and seen, for example, that 90% of people die within the first 11 months with a glioblastoma, I would've felt like, "I'm dead." Instead, never once did I think, *I'm not gonna make it.*

Today, I still have numbness. Overall my left side is a lot duller, and I have less control over it. Some brain-to-body connections have been broken by the surgeries. My big toe is just dead. I can't move my pinky or my ring finger on my left side, individually. I can only move them together. But I'm getting better. I've been doing physical therapy and occupational therapy every year since the surgery. I just keep going back. Insurance only gives me a certain amount of visits a year—I use them all up, then wait until the next year, then do it again. I'll never stop trying, because you just don't know.

I graduated from college in 2015. I had started in 2009. It took me a little while, because I was out of school for a year and a half during treatment. I didn't graduate with an early childhood education major, because I couldn't go back and work with the kids while I was in chemo and radiation. But I graduated with an educational studies major and two minors: sociology and nonprofit management.

I also started a hat-donation project called Gina's Journey in 2012, while I was in chemo. I wanted to be able to donate my hats to the hospital when my hair grew back, so others could use them. The Facebook page is www.facebook.com/GinasJourney/, and the husband of a teacher of mine made us a website: GinasJourney.org. We've been featured in local news and media. I collect hats, then get them dry-cleaned. I was turned down by two cleaners when I asked them to donate free dry-cleaning. Then I met Steve, whose daughter had cancer, and his dry-cleaning shop takes care of all of them. Once they're clean, I take the hats and put them in bins at the hospital. Anybody in the infusion centers, or the adult and pediatric cancer wards, can take any hat they want. Thousands of hats have been donated and taken by patients.

The Joy of Examination-Room Sex (And Other Sick Humor)

· ·

Name: Eileen Danial

Town: St. Clair Shores, Michigan

Diagnosis: Breast cancer; stage 2; HER2+

Age at diagnosis: 33

Age now: 35

At the University of Michigan Rogel Cancer Treatment Center, where I was treated for breast cancer, you start the ball rolling with an orientation where you meet all your doctors. On that day, I sat in the waiting room and looked around. At 33, I was the youngest person there. All the women seemed to be 50 and older—and there I was, in my Nike Dri-FIT shirt with yoga pants and gym shoes, thinking, *God, I can't wait to go for a run later with my boyfriend of a month, who has decided that he wants to stick around for this.*

That's Joe. We started dating a month before I was diagnosed; our anniversary is June 26th, and I was diagnosed July

> BEST ADVICE: You don't get a special award for handling the things that you handle. It doesn't make me less of a person or more of a person because I worked during cancer or during chemotherapy, took time off or didn't.

22nd. The day of my mammogram, I said, "I've got a doctor's appointment." We were in those early days, when you're just starting to discuss things that lead to trust. I said, "You know, I've got this lump in my breast, but I've had it before." I was just shrugging it off. I'd had noncancerous tumors removed when I was 18 and 19, so I wasn't that worried. I thought it might be the same issue, or maybe scar tissue from the surgeries. Joe listened, and his response was basically, "Just keep me posted."

A few weeks later, I was diagnosed. It was fast. At that point, I started trying to break up with him. I told him it wasn't fair and that he didn't sign up for this. He didn't have to do the noble thing by sticking around. If he left now, I could say it just didn't work out—and spare him from looking like the bad guy who dumped the cancer girl.

He let me babble on and on. Finally he said, "OK, well, you don't get to decide what I choose to do." That was huge for me, a turning point. I've always lacked true communication in relationships, and with him, it was totally different.

Joe joked, "All right, if we have to have a couple of dates at the clinic, then we have to." It's so funny. During the orientation, they leave you in this room for a couple of hours until the set of doctors can come in and see you. We were so young and new, and we flirted constantly. I said, "Man, we could totally get it on in one of these rooms." Of course, I wasn't really in the mood to be sexual or to make out in that room. "Hey, baby, we can convince someone to give us an extra hour once it's over." It was fun. Call it sick humor. From the beginning, joking was how I processed things; it was what I held onto during treatment, to remind myself and others that I hadn't lost *me* while I was sick. I told myself, I'm going through this, this illness, but this is not defining me or my life right now. It's part of a process.

Between Joe and me, inhibitions fell away immediately. We'd be sitting at these appointments where I'd have my shirt off and he'd be like, "Do you want me in the room or out?" I'm said, "At this point, everyone's seen it. Come on in."

I had two new giant things at once, cancer and this relationship. It was hard to experience the emotions specific to our relationship without bringing cancer into it. It was hard to know how to communicate things like, "I care about you—not because you're there for me, but especially because *you're* there for me." He's a great dude.

The first big treatment decision I made was to do a bilateral mastectomy. I had breast cancer in my family, and even before being tested for BRCA mutations, I knew that's what I wanted. My attitude was, *Just take both of them. I don't ever wanna worry about this again.* I have an obsessive nature, and I felt like I'd go through life always feeling the right one, looking for something. I also didn't want to have one real and one fake. I wanted the same thing on both sides.

After that, I met with the plastic surgeon and fell in love with him. He's an older man, and though of course he's a great and crazy-intelligent, that wasn't why. It was that he was so quirky and funny—exactly what I needed. Enough with the serious! (My oncologist, on the other hand—talk about serious. But I was fine with that. Save my life and we're good.) My plastic surgeon had funny ways to describe different procedures, like "rocks and socks" when describing implant profiles. He'd say, "Well, you don't want the rock-and-sock procedure, because that's what your boob will look like when we're done." He got me laughing. On that first day, when he drew out what he could do, he said, "God didn't get them perfect, so don't expect me to." He presented things in a way I could really relate to, and I think he got that I needed that.

We decided to do the mastectomy first, in September. Joe stayed the night with me at the hospital after the procedure and didn't leave until I was released. He was very involved and supportive, and he went out to get the meds I needed for recovery. I was very comfortable showing him my surgical scars when the nurse came over to help me shower. It didn't hurt that pain medication helps ease any tension you have! He never looked at me differently or felt pity. He just loved me through it all, even when I said I felt like a freak. We always shared how we felt, but he was never afraid—just always trusting the process, God, and my doctors.

I had 29 lymph nodes removed during the mastectomy, and 3 came back positive. That was scary for me. At first I thought it meant I was stage 4, but they explained that I fell into a gray area.

From the beginning, I read everything I could find. Knowledge is power. I thought if I could find everything there was to battle this, conventionally and holistically, then maybe I could help the next person do those things to heal themselves. Food became a tool, one thing that was easy for me to control. Right after I was diagnosed, I went on raw-vegan diet. But food was also a point of fear, because people said meat, sugar, or whatever else fed the cancer. Everyone suddenly becomes a certified oncologist when you have cancer, telling you what you should eat.

I took vitamin supplements. I met with a naturopath, on the recommendation of a friend I'd found who was 10 years out from her BC diagnosis. He put me on the supplements and had me juicing. Someone else recommended eating apricot kernels that I got online, for B17. I still have some and never want to take them again. They taste like bitter almonds, and I worked my way up to 20 a day. I was ready to try anything. If someone told me to stand on my head and drink a glass of water and recite the Declaration of Independence, I would've done it.

I knew I needed counseling, or some kind of emotional support from people like me who had gone through this. I tried one group where the youngest women were in their 60s and angry at the world. It was a bad match; I wanted to laugh, and they wanted to scream. I thought there had to be a support group for young women in my area. There's counseling for freaking everything, right?

I found the Young Adult Cancer Group, a.k.a. the Rack Pack, a local group for women under 40 dealing with any kind of cancer. I met a woman there, Sharon, who was just a couple of years older than me and had done the same chemo regimen that I was about to start. She drew up an outline and guidelines for me, describing everything she did and took to get through it. She said, "This all could happen to you, or maybe none of it will, but here you go. You're looking at me, and I'm alive." She was so inspirational to me, because she worked throughout her treatment and was doing so well. But then I met another woman who, poor thing, was just going through infections from her treatment, and hospitalizations and heart issues. Immediately I felt, "Oh, my God, they're gonna kill me." There's no happy medium in Eileen world. Either I was gonna do this in high heels or they were gonna kill me. All or nothing, always.

Finding the Rack Pack was such a relief, like I walked into the room and heard an *Ahhhhhhh* sound effect. That first day when it was my turn to share, I said something like, "Where the hell have you guys been?" Through them, I found out that with cancer come cancer perks—free camps like

Project Koru, a young-adult cancer camp offered for free to survivors thanks to scholarships, and retreats. There are so many foundations and activities that exist to help. The Pink Ladies of Charity send you care packages. Through the American Cancer Society, you can have someone come clean your house. Prosthetics were donated to me, but I didn't wear them. I had a year between my mastectomy and getting my expanders. I loved living in hoodies. It was the dead of winter. I was bald, constantly in beanies and hoodies. Hoodies fit better without boobs, so who really needed them? Being flat had its ups.

Sharon was the one who helped me figure out the sexual aspects of living with the disease. The doctors don't really talk to you about that stuff, but being in a new relationship, it was really important to me. I understand that vanity is one thing and feeling womanly another, but if cancer was going to strip me and make me vulnerable and bare, I wanted to own a part of *me* still. So Sharon and I had the girl talk. I could ask her questions like, "All right, so why am I dryer than the Sahara desert?" I was having Zoladex injections that put you into chemical menopause, a.k.a. chemopause—suppressing your ovaries helps protect your fertility later. But the hormones send you on an emotional ride. I'd ask Sharon, "Why can't I stand Joe right now? I can't stand him. Him breathing next to me makes me wanna stab him." Here's this poor, loving guy who's getting something new for me from the pharmacy for new side effects I have every five minutes, but I wanna kill him.

I had really long hair at the time. Before chemo, I got a bob, to start getting used to shorter hair. The first round of chemo was God awful. Every side effect that I could get, I got, including some really rare ones. I ended up with "adult acne meets chicken pox" all over my face and chest. Then add constipation, diarrhea, and bleeding, both rectally and vaginally. All of a sudden, I have this period that's not going away. Then nausea, mouth sores, dry mouth, and hair thinning. I started getting PTSD before the start of a new chemo cycle.

Joe was there for all of it—and when he couldn't offer solutions, he was there to listen, help me cope, and try to ease any worries or fears. He went on countless trips to CVS so I could try every lotion/anti-diarrhea/anti-rash/anti-constipation medicine he could find. If one thing didn't taste right, Joe made sure we had another option. He also took me for drives or walks just so I could get off the couch. He always reminded me I was beautiful—with or without adult acne, with or without hair, and with or without bleeding eyelids from eyelashes from falling out. He always made me laugh when I wanted to cry.

When the male pattern baldness started, I busted out clippers and shaved my own head. I owned that shit. I started to lose it up front instantly. I laughed about it, but I was also like, "No way am I gonna take this shit." My sister recorded me doing it, listening to music over the sink with $25 CVS clippers, cracking up: "Am I supposed to be emotional? Is something wrong with me right now? Oh, wait, I have cancer, so there's that." I had worried so much in the beginning about losing my hair that I was done with it. Give me a hat and a fun, colored wig. We're here, so I might as well look at it in the face and say, "All right. What's next?"

After chemo and a year of Herceptin, I had to decide whether to do radiation, which was optional but suggested for people in my gray area of one to three positive lymph nodes. I had a gut feeling that radiation was going to be bad for me. I told my thoughts to my plastic surgeon, and he supported me. He had been part of a study that suggested the cosmetic effects of radiation burns outweigh the benefits for people in the gray zone. If I'd decided to do it, reconstruction would have been a whole different ball game.

So I decided against it—the first thing I declined in my treatment. Sometimes family and friends, with and without cancer, made me feel ridiculed and shamed for my decision. You talk to people who seem to think, "I'm gonna do everything I can, whatever they tell me." Why? Doctors are human too. If something didn't feel right to me, I didn't want to do it. I felt that way about radiation, and I also felt that way about tamoxifen. I would not take one pill. Those are the two things that I declined, and I feel great about it still. Should anything happen, God forbid, should there be a recurrence, I have no regrets.

I did decide to try Nerlynx, which had just been introduced to the market. My insurance approved it, and the manufacturer of the drug assisted with the copay, so it was very affordable. I was told by the company who makes it that the drug is for women who have early-stage, HER2-positive breast cancer, have completed a year of Herceptin, and are within a two-year window of finishing that. I was also told it had a 34% rate of reduction of recurrence.

Let me tell you, I love marketing, *loooooove* marketing, everything about it—except pharmaceutical marketing when you're a cancer patient. All of their brochures give the 34% figure, which in the cancer world is fucking huge. You don't hear 34% in anything, besides the basic treatment. I thought, *Holy shit, 34% for a couple of pills for a year and maybe some diarrhea?* That was the only major side effect that was emphasized.

But Nerlynx was terrible. What a God-awful drug. I immediately ended up with nausea and a rash of red welts all over my chest, then a rash all over my chin, which I still have. Then came the mouth and throat sores. So now I have this yuck mouth which took me instantly to the PTSD of chemotherapy. I would rather have had the diarrhea all day long, every day, than that painful, burning mouth and throat. I couldn't eat anything, but I felt sick and knew I needed to.

I decided to quit it for good when I learned that 34% wasn't 34% but 2%. My plastic surgeon explained that the absolute or real effect is 2%, because the 34% just looks at women who took the pill in trial versus the ones who took the placebo. The real difference in recurrence is slight, because you have to consider what the likelihood of recurrence was for that specific pool of women, and then take the percent of the percent—which turns out to be 2. It became clear to me the risk was not worth the reward, should there even be one, since there's no long-term data to support it. Quality of life is where I'm at today. When it comes to my fear about quantity, that's what group therapy is for.

Sharing my experience about cancer with my broader circle of friends, people who didn't have cancer, was easier for me to do on Facebook than through text messages or email. I didn't feel like blogging. Facebook became a great outlet for me. Even in those posts, people could see I hadn't lost the wittiness and sarcasm that make me who I am—my true nature. Along with actual updates about my treatment, I'd write things like, "Hey, I haven't eaten in two weeks, but I've been binging the food channel." My saving grace was watching *Chopped* every night. I tried to have as much fun as I could and share that with the world, including wearing all the crazy wigs. I tried to make the best of a shitty situation.

The week before I went to Project Koru in Hawaii, Joe proposed. You know he wanted to make sure I didn't meet some cancer kid down there and fall in love! We got engaged, and we live together now. We have a house, and we just adopted a kitty. That's my joy, just every minute that I get to spend with them. Of course, as Joe reminds me, "You've only known the kitty for a week." I think I like him more than Joe does.

Fighting Lung Cancer in Public

Name: Jenna Gibson

Town: Sterling Heights, Michigan

Diagnosis: Lung cancer; stage 2; neuroendocrine carcinoid tumor

Age at diagnosis: 34

Age now: 39

In the movies, a doctor brings a patient into his office, seats her in a nice padded chair, sits down behind his beautiful mahogany desk, and then tells her the news that she has cancer. In my real life, I got a phone call at a little greasy-spoon diner called Ram's Horn, sitting across from my mom, trying to calm my four-year-old Anna and six-month-old Hope down while holding the waitress off. The room was spinning. I tried to write down everything that the PA said on a paper placemat, with a crayon, while holding back any tears from falling in the crowded restaurant.

That night, I had to go home and tell my husband. He's a very sentimental, emotional, kind-hearted man; I'm the strong, unbreakable one who never cries. He's a music pastor, so when I got home, I had to wait for band practice to finish; then I had to wait for the kids to go to bed. Finally, at 10:30 at night, sitting on the couch, he announces that he's tired and wants to go to bed. I said, "Well, so, there's one thing I wanted to talk about. I got a phone call today from the doctor."

Then I had to form the words to tell him that I had lung cancer. I can remember those moments very vividly—us in a quiet, dark room, a single lamp on. He asked me if he could pray with me. We're a very spiritual family, so I said, "Of course. Please do. Now more than ever." And then the jerk started to sing. Oh, my goodness. This man. For the first time since I got the

> WORST ADVICE: It's the same as the best advice. I believe that everything happens for a reason, and finding it helps you get through your days. But when you're going through this and somebody is telling you, "Everything happens for a reason," you just want to smack that person who doesn't know what you've been through and how you're suffering. It's not advice you can give to anyone. It is only advice you have to accept for yourself, when you're ready. God holds your future, and He will work all things for the good of those who love Him, but you have to put your trust in Him and let Him hold you through the pain. You may never know the reason, but being open to sharing your story will get you one step closer to helping someone else and fulfilling what your reason is.

news, I allowed myself to cry. I exploded into sobs.

That was two weeks before Thanksgiving, and I couldn't see the doctor until December 1st. He walked me through what would happen: "We're going to schedule your surgery. We're going to take your lung out. You're going to be in ICU for a number of days. We're going to get you up on the second day. You're going to have to cough a lot. We're going to walk you up and down the halls, and eventually we'll get you to a point where the chest tubes come out. And then you'll go home, and you'll be really tired." Some might say his delivery was sterile, but for me, he was so run of the mill about it all that I was reassured. I'm very much a planner, so I liked having it all laid out.

When he finished and asked if I had questions, I could barely get the words out to ask my biggest, scariest one: "Will my children get this?" But to this day, we have no idea. He thinks that a stem cell might have mutated as I was being formed in my mother's womb. Neuroendocrine carcinoid cancer cells can land anywhere, and mine happened to land and mutate in my lung. The tumor, which was the size of a tennis ball, was so calcified that he believed it was a very slow-growing, long-term thing. I had only discovered it through a fluke. It showed up during a routine health-assessment scan meant to kick off a weight-loss program. For more than a year—long enough for us to have our second daughter—doctors were sure it was benign. My beautiful daughter Hope is a miracle on so many levels. Had we known a year earlier that I had cancer, there's no way we would've ever had her.

I made my official announcement that I had cancer on Facebook on Christmas Eve—the first of many posts I made as I went through my illness. I lived my life in public there throughout my recovery and still to this day. "Finding out a few weeks ago that I have cancer is one of the scariest things I've ever had to face...Every last breath in my body exists for these girls to know how much Mommy loves them and for each person I meet to feel the love of Jesus through me. I will not let cancer take this from me."

I'm a strong Facebooker. I see it as a great tool to unite people. Without my support team there, of people all across the world, I don't know if I would have gotten through illness as well as I did. Posting there lead to people I haven't talked to since elementary school telling me they were supporting me, and how brave I was, and sharing stories with me. People have asked me to talk to their family members who are experiencing similar health challenges.

Surgery was scheduled for January 2015, and I decided I wanted to get a couple of things done beforehand. I wanted to get my youngest daughter's ears pierced, because it's something I did at six months of age. And I wanted to do family photos, because of course I thought, *This may be the last time*. It didn't look like I was going to make either happen, but then two days before the scheduled surgery, I got sick, so they postponed it until February 4. That's World Cancer Day, and it has been a very special day for me ever since. The postponement gave me the time I needed to do what I wanted. I was definitely a mess at JCPenney. I made the poor girl redo the photos a few times. I said, "Listen, I have cancer and I'll be having surgery next week, and these may be the last photos that my family will have of me—they have to be perfect!"

My mom and my husband posted all kinds of updates during and after my surgery, when I was groggy and out of it. It's cathartic for me to go back every year and relive those times. When the surgeon finished, my mother posted, "Surgery is over. All done through a scope-sized incision. Two-thirds of the right lung removed. The tumor was described as a 'large' tumor. The margins were clear. Several lymph nodes were biopsied. Now a three-day wait to get a definitive pathology report, to determine if further treatment will be necessary. Her vital signs are good. Hoping to see her in a few hours."

The next few days in the hospital were incredibly difficult. Unfortunately, the ICU was full, so I was in a group recovery room, behind a curtain, with an ICU nurse assigned to me. It was very uncomfortable. The next morning, the doctor came in to see me and talk to me, and he told me two things that were terrible news to me at the time. I was not allowed to drink any water, because I had so much fluid buildup from the surgery. I was incredibly upset about this because I was very dry-mouthed and thirsty. The second thing was that I had to continuously cough to get all the mucous and fluid out. It was so painful, and I was afraid I would bust a stitch. It hurt everywhere. It's like having a broken leg and being told you won't get better unless you walk on it.

I was in extreme pain. All I had going for me was the morphine pump, which I could only press every seven minutes. My husband's favorite story is that when he would come visit me, he would press the pump when I wasn't paying attention. I was expected to walk the hallways, but I had two chest tubes, a big machine that was suctioning the fluid out of my lungs through the chest tubes, and my IV pole. I couldn't walk well.

My mom was incredible. She is definitely an angel. When she was 18 years old, my grandmother sat her down and said, "You have two choices. You can either be a hairdresser or a nurse. Which one do you want to do?" And my mom picked nurse. Maybe she was meant to be a nurse for this reason, because there's no way I would have gotten through it all without her.

My mom spent every night with me while my husband took care of our sweet children. It was insane. But after three days, the physician's assistant came in to see me, and she said, "We got the pathology report back. Your margins are clear. We got all the cancer out, and I'm sending you home cancer-free." It was an amazing, unreal thing to hear. My husband took a great picture, and I posted on Facebook: "Going home as a lung cancer survivor, a little less lung, a lot more pain, and an incredibly thankful heart that Jesus has been fighting for me!"

I didn't require chemo or radiation; I was very lucky. But a week later, I went to my online patient account to read the pathology report. I was suddenly in shock when I read that they had found a different set of cancer cells in one of the bronchus tubes that was removed. Again, my head was spinning.

These cells were interpreted as precancerous small-cell carcinoma. At my next follow-up with the doctor, I asked him, "What the heck is this?" And he was dumbfounded, too. He is a highly regarded, respected thoracic surgeon. He said, "These are the type of cells typically found in a 70-year-old person who has smoked their entire life, not in a 34-year-old woman who's never smoked and who has just had a carcinoid tumor removed."

We sent the material out for a second opinion at the University of Michigan hospital. They classified it as a cell dysplasia, which is also interpreted as precancerous cells, whether inflammatory in nature or simply a disorganized cell type. The oncologist, a world-renowned specialist, told me he felt it the dysplasia was inflammatory. He said, "I would consider you 95% cured, and the 5% that's leftover is everyone's 5%."

Both doctors recommended yearly bronchoscopies along with six-month scans to keep an eye on it. Some days I feel like a ticking time bomb, but at other times, I just live like there's nothing more I can do. Now I'm on yearly scans. At some point in the next couple of years, I'll graduate to every two years, but eventually, there is a chance I'll get too much radiation from the scans. My doctor isn't used to having a patient so young.

I've only found three people with a diagnosis similar to mine. Unfortunately, the lung cancer community is very small and tight-knit because of the low rate of survivors over 5 years. The LUNGevity Foundation is the largest private funder of lung cancer research, and they sponsor different walks all across the country, as well as what they call "summits" in different cities nationwide. They have a major summit every April, the HOPE Summit. Over 300 survivors, caregivers, physicians, and oncology nurses come into Washington, D.C., to attend these educational seminars.

Three months after surgery, I was proud to complete the Breathe Deep Michigan 5K through the LUNGevity Foundation to raise money for lung cancer awareness and research. I walked very slowly, but I finished. It was amazing. My husband came with me, pushing our daughter Anna in the stroller. All of my fundraising was done through Facebook. I had a link to my story, which was shared through all my friends and family. Due to the amount of money I was able to raise, the LUNGevity Foundation sent me and my mom to the Hope Summit conference in Washington, D.C., for free. So we had a three-day weekend, conference tickets, and three nights in a hotel. It was fabulous. We even had some free time to visit various memorials in D.C.

We've gone a couple of times, but it's hard—you meet people and then those same people aren't always there the next year, because they haven't made it. I became very close with a few people that I've lost, and that was really hard for me. Losing one friend in particular was hard. She was pregnant and 26 years old, also a nonsmoker, when she was diagnosed with stage 4 lung cancer. She was a huge advocate, blogger, Facebooker—constantly trying to raise awareness. After about two years, her fight ended here on earth. I don't know how to say it. She didn't lose the battle. She battled *hard*.

I'm a very spiritual, faithful person. I have a strong belief in Jesus, and

I feel like I wouldn't be where I am without Jesus in my life. So I very much try to stick to my faith and not let fear grab hold. I'm also a compartmental-izer, and I have times when I just do not allow myself to think about things. It's a very sterile, cold place into which I lock my thoughts and fears, and I don't go near them. It's probably not healthy, but that's what I do, because I feel like I can't let fear own any part of me. I don't want to miss out on the joy—the time with my kids, my goofy husband, the events, the adventures. I may think about it, but I don't let it own me. I just lock it away.

I try to focus every day on things that matter. I like to say to my kids, and my mom, and my husband, "Let's go on an adventure." It can be anything spontaneous, like, "12 o'clock at night? Let's go grocery shopping. I don't care if we're in our pajamas. I want chocolate ice cream. Let's go to Taco Bell at 2:00 a.m." Let's just make every day something fun and exciting. Let's have things to look forward to. We're big believers, in my family, in not giving gifts but giving memories. So for Christmas, I may not give my mom a bunch of presents to open, but I always give her a memory—whether it's concert tickets, theater tickets, or an adventure somewhere.

The year after my surgery, we did a family trip to Disney World, an adventure to put the past behind us. I walked what felt like a number of steps that could break a Fitbit and was beyond any kind of physical tired I had felt before—because you know, lungs help! But the pain made me thankful. My husband talks about how pain is often like a receipt for the things that matter. When you miss someone you've lost, and it hurts, the pain is proof that you loved them and that it mattered. So, to me, the pain from walking and making it through the trip was good. The pain reminded me of how thankful I am, and now that pain has a sweet purpose.

My Daughter Saved My Life

Name: Jenn Korican

Town: Dexter, Michigan

Diagnosis: Breast cancer; stage 3; ER+, PR+, HER2+ ("triple positive"); invasive ductal carcinoma

Age at diagnosis: 34

Age now: 36

If I hadn't gotten pregnant with my daughter Riley, I don't know if I would have survived breast cancer. I call her my saving grace. Before I was diagnosed, in 2016, I was a full-time hair stylist at a salon in Ann Arbor. My first daughter was three. I had actually felt the lump in my breast for a year, but I was naïvely thinking, *Not me. It couldn't be me.* It hurt during my periods, so I thought it was one of those crazy period things. I had my mom feel it; I had my husband feel it. My mom wasn't concerned, because she said she got the same thing when she had her period and also had cystic breasts.

BEST ADVICE: This too shall pass, stay positive, and take it one day at a time. If you have a bad day, that's OK—just pick yourself up and don't stay in the dark hole for too long.

I probably would have continued to ignore it indefinitely, except that I got pregnant, and that changed the lump—one week later, it hurt so much I couldn't sleep on it. I couldn't even have a t-shirt or a tank top or anything on my breast, or I would wake up in sheer pain, crying. I didn't get in to see an OB until I was five weeks pregnant. Even though she wasn't concerned, we scheduled an ultrasound for the following week, since it's better not to have a mammogram while pregnant. I went thinking I was going to be in and out. Instead, they sat me down and said my lymph nodes were swollen, and they wanted to schedule a biopsy. That's when I started freaking out.

I went the next day for what was supposed to be a 90-minute appointment, but I was there for three and a half hours. They put a lead cape on me and did a mammogram first, of both breasts. Then they did a biopsy on the breast mass and one on my armpit. I got the phone call two days later. The doctor said, "I am glad that we did a biopsy, because the cells are compatible with cancer." He didn't give me any exact diagnosis. He just said a nurse navigator would be calling to set up appointments with oncology.

I was totally hysterical, cancelling my day's appointments and calling my parents, who cried with me. Later that afternoon I got a phone call telling me that I had the most common form of breast cancer, an invasive ductal carcinoma. When I later saw a doctor, I learned the pathology was "triple positive," which means they've identified three things that are fueling the tumor.

I knew so little at that point. I reached out to a friend who had been diagnosed a month before me and told her I was going down that same road, but also pregnant. She said, "I just read an article about a 21-year-old in Texas who has cancer and is pregnant and writing a blog." She gave me her name and encouraged me to get in contact with her. I found her on Facebook and sent her a private message. She responded after only an hour or so and was so positive. She said, "You can get through this. There is a group of us, the kick-ass cancer mamas. We've all been diagnosed during pregnancy with some form of cancer." She added me to the group, where I ended up getting a ton of support over the months, and answered every question I had.

Right away, the doctors told me I was their main concern—but in my heart, my baby was the main concern. Close family members, including my husband, also let me know that their first priority was me and that they would understand if we had to terminate the pregnancy. My father said, "We're not attached. We have to do whatever is best for you." I was a bit taken aback, thinking, *You might not be attached, but I am.*

At some point, my oncologist asked me, "Has anyone talked to you about termination?" I looked at her and I said, "Excuse me?" My husband said, "Would that change the course of her treatment or the survival outcome for Jenn?" She said no. "Then why would you even bring it up?" he asked. I looked at her square in her eyes, tears streaming down my face, and I said, "This baby saved my life. I'm going to do everything in my power to make sure that I get her here. She's worth it." The doctor nodded and said, "OK. I don't know what I would do in your situation, so I can't pass judgment."

From that point on, she knew that she wasn't just treating me but my unborn child as well. It was a lot of doctors talking back and forth. There were a lot of *what ifs* and *We don't knows.* I was a guinea pig, but I didn't care, as long as she was fine and I was still kicking cancer's ass.

The doctors told me that the CT scans I would need in the first trimester wouldn't be too much radiation for the baby. The breast surgeon recommended a unilateral mastectomy as soon as possible, followed by chemo while I was pregnant, then radiation after delivery. So at 12 weeks pregnant, I had a unilateral mastectomy, with 21 lymph nodes removed. When I learned that all the lymph nodes were positive, meaning they could have pumped that cancer anywhere in my body, I was sure I would never live to see my daughter's first birthday.

I started chemo at about 16 weeks. The first cycle was Docetaxel, Carboplatin, and Herceptin. I was going in biweekly to do fluid checks for the baby. With the Herceptin, the drawback was it would take a toll on my kidneys; therefore I wouldn't have a lot of amniotic fluid. It became a constant battle with this fluid. There were days when there was some, and there were days when there was hardly any. They sent me to triage to get monitored because there wasn't a lot of fetal movement. There came a point where we stopped the Herceptin for a couple of weeks, then tried again on half doses, then just stopped it altogether because of the danger to the baby.

At that point, I was doing weekly fluid checks. They were trying to do anything to keep her in there as long as they could. At 25 weeks I went in for an appointment, and the doctor had trouble finding a fetal count, so she sent me to triage. They gave me some steroid injections and said, "You might be having this baby sooner than you think."

From 26 weeks on, I went to three or four doctors appointments a week, up until I delivered at 36 weeks. I was going every other day to get a stress test or an NST, and then when I wasn't getting NSTs, I was getting ultrasounds. I was just at the doctor all the time, until I delivered Riley on June 12, 2017.

After delivery, I did radiation. Then I went back on Herceptin and also Perjeta, until January of 2018. The Perjeta was terrible. "Never trust a fart" is what I said on Perjeta. It was bad.

Reconstruction wasn't an option for me because they'd removed so much tissue, so my breast surgeon gave me a "knit knocker." There's a community of ladies that make these little crocheted boobs stuffed with cotton for cancer centers. More recently, I got a prosthetic.

I haven't been back to work. It feels like this is an opportunity for me to stay home with my girls and be present. We're making memories. I'm on an aromatase inhibitor and oral chemo now, and I'm having the problem that I worry about every little ache, pain, lump, and bump. The women in my support group told me about the two-week rule.

WORST ADVICE: Lemon's cure cancer!! Wow, really??? Then nobody should have cancer.

If it's still there or if you still feel that pain after two weeks, then call your doctor and make an appointment. I try to tell myself not to get caught up in everything. The majority of my friends now are cancer survivors.

Unfortunately, in a group of women with so many different forms of cancer, I've seen many go. It's hard. I have to tell myself it's not my story. That's not my diagnosis, that's not me. But it's hard because you make such strong bonds with these women, even the ones you never meet in person. We all went through it, so we know how to help each other.

My joy is trying to help other women going through what I went through. If telling my story saves one person or helps one woman, that's what matters to me. Shortly after I delivered, one of my doctors reached out to me through Facebook and said that they had a patient referred to them who was pregnant and just diagnosed with breast cancer. She didn't want a support group; she didn't want to go talk to anyone. But when the doctor brought me up, the lady just started crying. The doctor said, "Would you like me to see if she can get in contact with you?" She was overjoyed. We eventually got on the phone, and I knew it meant so much to her to talk to someone who had been through it and delivered a healthy baby.

Riley is now 21 months old, and she is absolutely amazing! I may be partial as her mom, but she communicates so well and says far too many words. You can have a full- fledged conversation with her. Right now her favorite food is "cado." She will eat avocado for breakfast, lunch, and dinner. We have outgrown highchairs at restaurants, because she would prefer to be in a booth like a big girl. We just went on our first vacation as a family of four. It was intense but amazing. It brought me and my girls so much closer.

Celebrating with a Half Marathon

Name: Tami Langenright

Town: Milan, Michigan

Diagnosis: Hodgkin's lymphoma; stage 2

Age at diagnosis: 34

Age now: 36

W hen I was diagnosed, my husband and I were living in our first home together, a condo we had purchased a little over a year before. We both worked for the local county government, me in human resources. We were just working and enjoying life. We were thinking about kids in the future, but for the present, we wanted to enjoy our life together and travel.

It took months of doctors and tests and feeling sick before I got my diagnosis. I had to keep pushing—I knew something was wrong with me. I had a bunch of symptoms, including pinkeye, rashes, stomach issues, and swollen lymph nodes, but not the classic ones, like night sweats, that would have screamed "cancer."

BEST ADVICE: Follow your gut instincts. When I was starting to feel weird symptoms, I could have just said, "Oh, OK, it's probably not a big deal." But I knew that there was something wrong. I knew that it was not normal. So I kept going back to the doctors, and I didn't give up until I had an answer I was satisfied with.

Finally, they did a biopsy. The doctor called and said it didn't look like cancer but that there were necrotic cells, which meant something was eating away at my lymph nodes. So they were going to send me to a disease specialist, kind of like a "Dr. House," to try and figure out what was going on. We were texting our friends and our family, who were rejoicing that it wasn't cancer. But I thought, *Oh my God. It's something worse than cancer. What is happening? What's inside my body? What is this?*

A day or two later, the doctor called me again at work. I share an office with a woman named Sarah, who is an amazing friend. I thought the doctor was calling with info about the specialist. Instead he said, "I have really bad news for you. We had other pathologists look at the stains, and I was, in fact, wrong. It is classic Hodgkin's. All I can do is ask for your forgiveness and tell you how sorry I am."

I hung up the phone and looked at Sarah. I said, "That was the doctor, and they were wrong. I have Hodgkin's. I have cancer." And then I just completely lost it. We shut the door, but my boss could see that I was crying through the little windows. She came in, and I couldn't even talk. Sarah had to tell her. My boss was just hugging me as I sobbed. And then I was like, "I gotta go. I gotta go to Mike. I can't call him. I have to go to his work. I have to go." They offered to drive me, but I knew driving would calm me down.

At Mike's work, I texted him: "You need to come outside right now." When I told him, he looked lost. I've never seen him look like that before, like he didn't know what to do. That was a really rough day. From there, it got better, I guess. Better and worse.

I remember being really afraid of what treatment would be like because of what I had seen on TV and in movies. The person is really, really sick, throwing up all the time, and really sickly looking. That scared me. My oncologist assured me right away: "There's tons of medicine out there, so you should never feel sick. You should never throw up." Now I get so mad when I see something that is not really accurate to what the experience is like.

I was also so afraid of losing my hair. I had long, curly hair; it was my one physical pride. I had to sign a statement before my first chemo treatment that said I was going to be treated for something that could kill me—and that the drugs I was receiving were deadly and could also kill me. So maybe worrying about my hair was a defense mechanism. It was easier for me to obsessively worry about that than to worry about dying.

People told me, "Yeah, but you'll get to wear fun wigs" or "It's just hair; it'll grow back." Those comments weren't at all helpful. First of all, I never wore wigs because they're uncomfortable, and not everybody has the confidence to pull that off. I did not want to draw attention to myself. I'm not someone who's going to show up to work at my human-resources job wearing a fluorescent-orange or blue wig. Everybody goes through their own kind of journey. I know people were trying to be encouraging and supportive, but for me, that was probably not the best thing to say.

The beginning of my treatment and leading into it was a whirlwind. My husband would catch me staring off into the distance, especially when we drove home after appointments. He would ask, "What are you thinking right now?" And I would say, "Nothing really." I was just in a numb, weird, blank state sometimes.

I started focusing on the next immediate step in front of me. Like, "OK, I got the PET done. I got through that horrible experience." And then, "Now I have to get my port installed. Once I get the port installed, then I have to do the pulmonary-function test. And I have to get the heart test done, to make sure that my heart and my lungs can handle the chemo. OK, we got that done. Now we gotta go for the first chemo." If I focused on the whole picture, it was too overwhelming.

My chemo treatments were every other Thursday. On the day of my treatments, I would get my blood taken. I would see my doctor or my nurse, and then I would do my chemo. So I would take Thursday and Friday off work, recover over the weekend, and then go to work either Monday morning or afternoon.

I had already gone through most of my sick time in the process of getting diagnosed. But my job allowed coworkers to donate their sick time to me. My coworkers donated enough that I didn't have to worry about unpaid leaves of absence for doctor appointments or treatments. My husband, Mike, was by my side every single step of the way. There was only one appointment that he missed. He works for the same local government, and they were very helpful in making that possible.

The amazing support from our very large network of close friends and family made everything easier. They were always visiting. They did a meal train, so we had coworkers and friends that we hadn't seen in years dropping off meals for us. People sent cards and donated money. Mike's aunts own a bakery. One of my favorite cookies is macarons, and they learned how to make them and did a fundraiser for me. Every single person that came in to buy macarons, the money went directly to us. There was a huge outpouring of love and support. Being sick was a horrific experience, but at the same time, it was an amazing experience to receive all of that love.

When I went for the first meeting with my oncologist, he said the chemo I would be getting doesn't typically affect the ovaries but that it was better to take precautions. I didn't have enough time to freeze my eggs, which was fine. Mike and I were still on the fence about children, and I don't think either of us was really ready. But I was interested in the Lupron injection, which basically shuts down your ovaries and hides them so the chemo doesn't attack them. As part of that process, I saw a fertility specialist, who tested my ovarian function.

The next day, I got a call from her. (Over time, I learned that it's not usually the best-case scenario when you see a doctor's number pop up after testing.) She said, "I hate to make these phone calls, but I have bad news. You have pretty much no ovarian functionality. So not only do I recommend you getting the Lupron injection, but if you ever were to decide to have children, the chances of you being able to have them without medical intervention are 0-to-5%." Not only did I find out that I have cancer, but then I found out I most likely could never have children.

My best friend, Courtney, ordered rubber bracelets from the Leukemia and Lymphoma Society and sent them to all of my friends, family, and coworkers, with a letter, before my first treatment. The instructions were to flood my Facebook and my text messages with well wishes and love during my first treatment and the rest of the treatments after. So while the first treatment was incredibly scary, all those messages kept me distracted from the fear. It made me so happy to see all the love and support coming in.

What I found the hardest about the experience wasn't what I expected. Like I said, I thought it would be throwing up, looking sick, and losing my hair. But something I had never thought about, or heard about, turned out to be the hardest thing: There are so many things you're not allowed to do. I couldn't eat at potlucks. I couldn't eat from salad bars. I couldn't eat cold subs. If I went out to eat, I couldn't go at prime time. It had to be when the restaurants were a little empty. If we went to the movies, we had to make sure we weren't sitting close to anybody. I couldn't go grocery shopping. I couldn't clean up after our pets. I couldn't really clean, energy-wise. I was neutropenic almost immediately, so if I was around anybody who was a little bit sick, I could get super-sick—and it could send me into the hospital and possibly kill me. I didn't go out to concerts or into really full public areas for seven months. (I was in treatment for six months, but I was neutropenic for a month after my last treatment.) All those little things that you never think about really add up.

Another big surprise of cancer was more positive: It lead to me running my first half marathon. This started because one of my very close friends, Heidi, was a runner. When I got sick, she felt the need to do something. She signed up for the Detroit Free Press full marathon to raise money for the Leukemia and Lymphoma Society.

She ran the marathon shortly after I was done with treatment. I got to go and cheer her on. While I was there, I looked at all the runners. Some of them were not in the best shape. Some were really young. Some were really old. I was seeing all different types of people. I started thinking, *Wouldn't it be awesome if one of them were me?* The whole past year, I had been in treatment. How amazing would it be if this year I trained! Instead of six months of chemo, I'd do six months of training and run a half marathon.

The anniversary of my diagnosis was hard for me. I really struggled. So I wanted to make sure that the anniversary of my first treatment was different. That day, I signed up for the half marathon. I started raising money for the Leukemia and Lymphoma Society, and I started training—the first time, literally in my life, that I'd stuck to a workout regimen. I'd finish a really hard run and think, *A year ago I was getting my sixth chemo treatment, and now I'm running. I'm struggling to breathe, and I feel like I want to quit—but a year ago, I would have given anything to do this.* That awareness kept me going.

In October, I ran the half marathon with my husband. He had trained with me the entire time without knowing whether he'd run. Heidi ran, too—along with one of our other lifelong friends, Jason, and my officemate and close friend, Sarah. Sarah's dad even ran with us! Some of our friends showed up and cheered us along. It was an amazing experience.

Running the half marathon was incredibly therapeutic and, I think, helped me in more ways than I could have realized. Mike and I have truly learned how to enjoy life, let the little things go, and focus on what's important to us. It has been hard trying to find the positive in cancer and chemo treatments. My first year in remission was hard. I think I was still in the "feeling angry and resentful" phase.

But today, so much has changed—and one big thing in particular. I am currently 18 weeks pregnant with a very healthy baby boy. We had considered fertility treatments, but my ovaries surprised us, and it happened naturally. I'm pregnant and thriving.

A Self-Authored Approach to Healing

Name: Ali Marie Shapiro

Town: Pittsburgh, Pennsylvania

Diagnosis: Hodgkin's lymphoma; stage 2

Age at diagnosis: 13

Age now: 40

Even though I was diagnosed 26 years ago, I still vividly remember my emotional state at the time. It doesn't leave you, however long it's been. I was coming to the end of my seventh-grade year, and I wanted to get in shape for a middle-school dance. It seems so innocent now. My dad had this thing called the NordicTrack. In Pittsburgh, the weather is good for three days a year, so you have indoor exercise equipment. I was trying to get my heart rate up, and I took my pulse in my collarbone area, which is where I thought your pulse was. That's how much I knew about my body. I found a lump there. My dad took me to the doctor, and I was scheduled for a biopsy within the week.

BEST ADVICE: As soon as you're done with the curing part of your protocol, you gotta figure out how to heal. There's a radical difference between curing and healing. No matter how much you might get dismissed by the traditional system, go find the resources to help you heal. They're out there for you.

I got the news as soon as I woke up from surgery. The surgeon came in and said, "I have good news and bad news. What do you want first?" I wanted the bad news first. He said, "It's cancer." It was almost like time suspended. I heard him saying this, and I looked over and saw my parents. I had never seen my dad cry before, but he was crying. Then I knew it was real. The doctor continued, "The good news is that this is Hodgkin's disease, which has an 80% cure rate." I had this weird feeling of *I'm going to die* and *I'm going to live*, at the same time. My life was never the same.

I had six straight months of chemo, a month off, then a month of radiation. I got a Mediport to stop my veins from collapsing. Radiation, when it came around, felt like a piece of cake for me compared to chemo.

I didn't know this at the time, but I am part of the first generation of childhood cancer survivors who survived en mass. The generation before me had treatment that didn't work as well. When I was treated, in terms of long-term care, there were not a lot of frameworks to follow—just uncertainty. You're followed for five years after. What I found out, over the course of many years of health struggles following my treatment, was that Western medicine had been great at curing me from Hodgkin's but was completely unequipped to help me heal in the aftermath.

In the years after I was cured, I struggled physically and emotionally. Cancer disorients you. Anything you believe about the world basically disintegrates—at least, I felt that way. My mom is into reincarnation, but my dad is agnostic. He says he believes in nature. I always wondered what came after death, even before I got sick. I didn't have a religious compass. I didn't have a philosophical compass. After my diagnosis, I felt no sense of order at all.

Having cancer so young was deeply emotionally traumatizing, and that ultimately affected my physical health—but it took me more than a decade to understand that. I wanted to be normal. I wanted to pretend nothing had happened, and I was flooded with people saying, "You're so strong." You often feel like you have to be strong for other people because they're devastated as well.

My unresolved trauma manifested, at first, in food and weight issues. First I got really into exercising. When you're 14, because of our culture, you think being healthy is being skinny, so in my mind I was getting healthy. I maintained a really low weight and didn't have many health problems. Then I went to college, a huge transition. If you have unresolved trauma, those big, uncertain transitions become triggers. I blew up into an emotional eater and a binger.

I started trying different therapists. I got on four or five antidepressants, having no idea that my gut was destroyed—not just from the chemotherapy and the steroids, but dear God, from the emotional stress as well. I started having more and more health issues. I was diagnosed with Irritable Bowel Syndrome (IBS). My asthma and allergies were escalating. I had gone on Accutane and different antibiotics for my skin previously, and all those issues came back.

When you go through cancer, your doctors become like God. They were for me. It was like, "Oh my God, whatever you tell me to do, I'm going to do it." That saved my life. But by my early 20s, their protocols were no longer working for what had become chronic issues. The doctor was prescribing meds that weren't working. For years, I had defined being healthy as not having cancer. I didn't have cancer anymore, but I was not healthy either. I was really struggling.

Over time, I learned that my binge eating and depression weren't independent diagnoses—they were symptoms of my real problem, the fact that I hadn't processed the emotional side of being sick and facing death at such a young age. Anyone who goes through something hard in our culture faces this problem. "Toughness" is promoted as carrying on and sucking it up. Being strong. Instead, we need to be able to say, "This has forever changed my life, and I have to face it. I have to face that I can't go back to where I was. How am I going to move forward in a way that can make the pain I've gone through count?"

My story isn't so unusual. Many of us who go through cancer end up struggling with chronic issues like depression, anxiety, asthma, or IBS. All of these are chronic issues that the American health-care system was never designed to address. It's focused on treating acute disease, and it excels at that. Once you understand that healing afterward requires something else, you can reorient. There are amazing doctors doing amazing things within the traditional health-care system, and I don't want to dismiss that. But being well and trying to fight disease are just very different things.

In trying to heal my physical self, I found my way to the Institute for Integrative Nutrition, and ultimately I received my certificate in partnership with Columbia University's Teachers College, which was associated with the center at the time. Over time, I learned to look at food not as good or bad, but as medicine. I took the shame out of it. I found out I was gluten intolerant and started taking probiotics. I thought the food I was eating was healthy, but most of it was packaged. Some basic changes really turned my health around. After two years of learning about holistic nutrition for my own needs and clearing up issues my doctor's weren't able to resolve, I realized, "Oh, my God, people need to know about this. I need to share this."

I spent about a year working with clients in addition to my corporate job. I had my health-coaching certification and started out by giving people grocery-store tours to help them get off packaged, processed food. This was radical 12 years ago. But soon, I realized that by the fourth session, we weren't talking about food anymore. I thought, *If I'm going to be able to help these people, I'm going to need more education.*

Then I entered grad school. I actually got my master's at the University of Pennsylvania. I started studying the change process and coaching. It sent me down a rabbit hole of how we learn and the mindsets that we bring to things. I don't mean mindset like, "You gotta think positive." I mean the actual way that we make meaning. To heal, I learned to shift—and eventually, to help my clients shift—from being a passive patient to being an active advocate. We have to trust ourselves and our ability to do that. There have been times when I've had to challenge my doctors—and sometimes leave doctors because I'm feeling dismissed.

As a cancer survivor, being a self-advocate is a lot harder than it sounds. You have a learned mindset: "I can't trust my body. It failed me. I got cancer." To change that, we need to relearn how to become what the research calls *self-authoring*. I call it "the boss mindset." You take control of the narrative and change the meaning of what has happened to you. I wanted to create a process to help people make that shift, from passive patient to self-authoring advocate.

To change is to heal. I could see that so many people were missing out on the opportunity to make the most of the pain we've gone through. I've come to believe that true healing happens when we make our pain count, when we make a reason for it. For me personally, I'm healing myself by helping other people with their path to wellness. I spent 4 1/2 years in grad school, developing and refining my process. What I realized is, a lot of these change processes focus on our thoughts and the mental piece of this—but when you've gone through trauma, there is emotion lodged in your nervous system. You need to focus on the heart and the head for lasting change. You have to come out of the world with a different way of seeing it. That's a lot easier said than done.

The result of all this work is my program, Truce with Food. I really like Eastern philosophy and Eastern thought—but I'm a Western person, so I wanted a framework to basically prove the Eastern wisdom. The program at first was six weeks. We did it in person in Philadelphia. It has grown and evolved in the nine years since I began. I'm now certifying Truce with Food to coaches, doctors, nurses, and anyone who can use it to help people heal.

At the heart of healing is learning to trust life again. I wanted to create a framework that didn't tell people what to do but helped them to trust themselves—basically, what I wish I'd had all those years ago. It took me twelve years to get healthy. Looking back, it's ridiculous, especially when you consider how much privilege and incentive I had. Imagine how people with less resources, access, and support fare.

My own health journey continues. As I heal, I find myself enamored with the ordinary, which to me is extraordinary. I don't have to set an alarm in the morning. For so many years in the corporate world, I had to get up, work out, get my breakfast, rush to work. I feel so much joy. I love being with my clients. Also, we just got my first dog ever. It was my husband's idea. Being with him and watching him is hilarious to me.

It took twelve years, but I found a way to make my pain count. I help people understand and heal their trauma and, in the process, their bodies. To see them step into their power and get to a place where they can take advantage of the capacity they've developed by going through so much difficulty—that really gets me up in the morning and gives me joy.

Stand-up Comedy to Release the Rage

· ·

Name: Emily Strong

Town: Inver Grove Heights, Minnesota

Diagnosis: Breast cancer; stage 3; ER+, PR+, HER2+ ("triple positive")

Age at diagnosis: 33

Age now: 37

When I was diagnosed, I was on the tail end of "babyland." I'd had my daughter 19 months prior and was starting to get my body back and feeling good. At work, I had taken on a new and challenging role. I was getting sleep! Our little family was healthy and growing...or so I thought. What I didn't know was that I had been growing something else—a whole lotta breast cancer.

The doctor who told me "You definitely have cancer," in the most cavalier manner during an ultrasound, was not sympathetic in any way. He struck me as a kind of hair-plugged, Ferrari-driving, hotshot kind of guy. As I lay sobbing on the exam table, he patted me awkwardly on my naked shoulder and mumbled a robotic, "It'll be OK. We'll take good care of you." It was a surreal experience, and I felt lost and out of control.

BEST ADVICE: *Do not* immediately assume you are dying. Your first step is not death— your first step is treatment. And the whole point of treatment is to make you better. So don't wallow in the "fact" that you're gonna die. Cancer isn't a death sentence.

All the steps and appointments leading to this moment should have been clear signs that something was wrong. I feel foolish now not to have caught the level of concern from my primary-care doctor and the urgency with which she scheduled my mammogram. I went in one day from mammogram to ultrasound to biopsy. I woke up that day thinking, *What if?...Nah!* and ended it on the floor in my husband's arms, just screaming and sobbing and screaming some more. I was convinced I was going to die.

Between my initial tests and finally seeing a doctor, I had to wait two weeks. It was two weeks of crying and "Dr. Google" (which, as an aside, I do *not* recommend). I was that patient who constantly called the oncology department for more information—for fucking answers! Finally, the staff took pity and got a nurse practitioner to talk to me. She set my expectations and made me feel like all I would need was medication...nothing major. She said I probably wouldn't even need chemo.

The longest two weeks of my life passed, and I had my appointment with a real, live doctor. I had the last appointment of the day, at 3:00 p.m. The nurse led me back to the exam room—and she kept crying. She tried to hide it, and I asked if she was OK. She nodded and quickly excused herself from the room. It seemed weird that she was crying, but I thought maybe she'd had a hard day or something. So I sat there in my gross little gown thing, joking with my husband while flipping through the American Cancer Association's wig catalogue. It was straight out of 1989! Those were some sweet do's. There was a "Princess Diana," and these things called "wisps" that you could clip under your hat or scarf as if they were lady sideburns (I mean, how would those things hide the fact that you were bald?). Thinking back now, it's strange the details that stick out…but at the time, those glued-on hair things were hysterical.

Finally, the doctor came in and immediately launched into her spiel about "starting chemo right away, in a week or two" and "Oh, you should get a port—all my patients love their ports." Now remember, the last thing I'd heard was I likely wouldn't need chemo. Other than that, I really hadn't received any information since Dr. Hair Plug had dropped the big "C-bomb" on me. I had a pen in my hand that I had planned to use to take notes, but instead I screamed "FUUUUUUUUUCK!" and threw the pen so hard that it stuck in the wall. This was clearly not the reaction the doctor had expected, and she froze. A polite but urgent knock on the door signaled that I had made an impression outside the exam room. The doctor realized that I hadn't been properly prepped, and she apologized. Apparently, I was supposed to receive a call that would prepare me with more information—but I hadn't. After the appointment ended, a mere 90 minutes later, the nurse who had been crying rushed up to me and, still crying, hugged me, saying, "You are so beautiful, and nothing, not this cancer, not anything, will make you any less." It was obvious to me then that she had been crying because my prognosis was so upsetting.

Everything happened quickly once I met with my oncologist, a grumpy and slightly condescending older man. He reviewed my information and provided a formal diagnosis: stage 3A breast cancer—HER2 positive, estrogen-receptor positive, and progesterone-receptor positive. Shortly after that, I got my port placed, and two days later it was "chemo class" and my first infusion. I had four rounds of chemo, a double mastectomy with expanders, six more rounds of chemo, 35 sessions of radiation, and finally, reconstructive surgery.

When I look back, I remember that I was so, so very angry. The fear manifested into rage. The steroids I took prior to each infusion didn't make my mental situation any better. I was angry this was happening to me. I was angry that I had to lose my hair. I was angry that I couldn't have estrogen—that I'd gain weight and sleep poorly, my lady bits would dry up, my skin would look terrible. Most of all I felt utterly, horribly guilty. I didn't deserve to be loved; it would have been better if I hadn't married and had my children. I just remember thinking, *Who can I scream at about my diagnosis? Who can just sit there and take it?*

I was really open about my feelings with family and friends. I wanted to help them understand that breast cancer wasn't just "fluffy pink shit" and long-ass walks to raise awareness and money. I spoke honestly when people asked me how I was doing. I posted treatment updates along with my feelings on my CaringBridge health blog. I'd get the overused "Just stay positive!!!!!" and the "Have you thought about seeing someone?" I did think about my mental health, a lot. I knew that I needed to talk to an impartial person and unload my rage, fear, despair, and self-loathing on someone who could carry it. My hospital provided an inept therapist who was barely my age and repeated the "stay positive" BS. She kept telling me I was "beautiful without hair." I was quick to eliminate her from my care team and spent nearly eight months trying to find a therapist who could help me.

Ultimately therapy, an antianxiety medication, time, and eventually humor gave me perspective and a bit of peace. Coming to grips with the new reality of my life was the hardest part. Until all of my treatments wrapped up, I, myself, hadn't done much. The medical pieces of treatment were easy—I wasn't doing anything; science was healing me. I felt like such a fraud as everyone kept telling me I was brave and awesome. I knew I had to do something brave and awesome, something that was totally me, that would help me "own" this experience. I wanted to physically demonstrate that all of this wasn't about what cancer took from me but what I gained.

As I was recovering from my reconstructive surgery, I received an email from ACME Comedy Club, a local joint I adore. The club was hosting their annual "Funniest Person" contest and looking for contestants. I was like, *Heck yeah! I'm gonna register, I'm gonna do it, and it's gonna be awesome!* I had done public speaking and presentations where I used humor to communicate, but I had never done pure stand-up. When I saw that email, I immediately submitted an application to perform a few months later. That same evening I got an email back from the club… *I was in!*

Honestly, I am an 11th-hour kind of gal. I'd jot down funny things here and there, collecting bits I thought would make a fine set. As I got closer to my performance, I realized I had way more material than I had time to deliver. A few nights before the actual competition I sat on the floor of my bedroom, locked the door to prevent children from interrupting, and had a moment of what I consider pure genius. I had the perfect comedy act.

The night of the show was absolutely wonderful. I had a huge, badass crowd of supporters who raised the roof with their cheers. I felt so powerful, so in control. I was making people laugh, and I was using my experience to demonstrate that I was not fucking broken; I was not fucking dead. I was alive, radiant, and hilarious.

I had spent eight months going through hellish treatments that altered my body, mind, energy, and relationships. In those moments that I stood on that stage, bald-headed, bawdy, and beautiful, making people laugh while sharing my anger, it all seemed worth it.

I don't want to imply that one night of stand-up comedy made my experience with cancer all O.K. It surely didn't. I still bear the emotional and physical marks of how this has altered my life forever. But turning all that garbage I had gone through into comedy helped me acknowledge the anger and trauma for what it was—and to realize that what *I* am is still very much ahead of me.

I also need to stress the importance of my enormous support network of family and friends, and especially my spouse, who held me up when I couldn't or just didn't want to cope. I did none of this on my own, and I really credit the people closest to me as my saviors. They let me rage, and they rallied a veritable army for me before each infusion, each surgery, and my return to work. My mom put it best: "We'll clear the runway so Emily can land the plane."

Before cancer, I spent a lot of time focusing on my appearance and how others viewed me. The perspective of age, paired with this experience, has shown me that I am so much more than my physical form. Even with fake, lumpy boobs and many extra pounds, I feel better about who I am and what I do. I finally get what "living in the moment" means, and I actively focus on appreciating what I have while I plan for the future.

The whole time I've known my husband, he always has said to me, "It doesn't matter what you look like. It doesn't matter what you achieve. I will always love you. I am here because of you. And we have this family because of you. And as long as you're in it, everything's gonna be OK." I don't think I ever really got it until I went through this. Now, when I put my head in "my spot" on his shoulder, I feel peace and can let go of my rage.

Blogging with Vulnerability, Accepting Support

Name: Shelly Vaughn

Town: Munroe Falls, Ohio

Diagnosis: Breast cancer; stage 2

Age at diagnosis: 36

Age now: 39

I'm not naïve about the world of cancer. I've lost friends and family to the disease. My mom has stage 4 breast cancer. I always knew there was a chance I'd be diagnosed, but I never dreamt it would be so soon in life.

I was living my life as a wife and mother, with two lovely girls who were 7 and 9 years old. I was working full-time as a speech-language pathologist and playing volleyball a few times a month. I would say I had a very fun, active lifestyle. Our family was always out doing things—hiking, kayaking, biking, going to museums and festivals. The girls were busy taking dance classes, cheerleading lessons, and piano lessons. I had always been a very healthy person. But there was no denying the lump I felt on my own one day.

As soon as I felt it, my heart sank. Though I prayed it was benign, it just didn't seem right. I got into the doctor as soon as I could; I was referred to a surgeon and then to another doctor for a biopsy. On Friday, January 20, 2017, I got the dreaded phone call at work.

"Lisa" was the woman from my surgeon's office who called. She said the words "invasive, poorly differentiated ductal carcinoma"—and my brain could barely process what she was saying. She repeated it, and I needed her to spell out the words to know what they were. Even then, I stared at the yellow post-it note, in disbelief that this was my information. Those words were describing what was in my body. My whole world stopped making sense that day.

I called my husband, Rob, right away. It was such a hard phone call to make. He immediately came to my office and held me while I cried, not knowing what to say and barely knowing what to do next. That was the beginning of my witnessing that the man I married was not only amazing in all the ways I had previously known, but he was also amazing in the role as my caregiver.

Rob stayed with me while I called my twin sister, Trisha, then as I called my close friend who would pick up our girls from the bus stop that day and take them to dance class. We had to get to another appointment now, the first of so many appointments, to learn about this disease that would change my life.

Hearing devastating news is hard, but sharing it with loved ones makes you relive that shock over and over again. And there's not much worse than knowing that your phone call is about to ruin someone's day. My sister drove to Ohio from Pennsylvania that afternoon and helped me make the initial calls to tell my parents, brother, and close friends. I tried to tell some people myself, and it was really hard. They would cry, which would make me want to cry. I would try to be strong and tell them it was okay, which was not easy to do when I was struggling to believe that myself.

We have a huge extended family, and there was no way I could repeat those difficult conversations multiple times. Looking ahead, there were going to be so many appointments and updates almost daily for the first few weeks, and I needed to figure out a way to keep everyone updated and current. I was worried that I would forget who I told what information to. Would I forget to tell my family something that I shared with people at work? So many people would be praying for me, but how could I make sure they knew what specific prayers we needed?

My husband is actually the one who suggested that I start a private Facebook group. It was the perfect solution for me. I'm on Facebook anyway, and I knew most of my family and friends were, too. I started the group the next day and called on a few close girlfriends to help me come up with a name for it. I used a special photo of my husband as the cover photo. As trivial as it may seem, keeping my mind focused on details with the Facebook page helped distract me from thinking about cancer growing inside of me. I also felt really comfortable sharing my personal information in that controlled space.

BEST ADVICE: Don't assume longevity. None of us, at age 6 or 36 or 76, know how much longer we'll be around. But for some reason we all assume we'll live long enough to turn gray, retire, hold grandbabies, and watch the sunset from our rocking chairs (Do people really do that?). I remember a "longevity calculator" online told me once I'd live until 92. Yep—that sounded about right. That's exactly what I was thinking. But now I realize how silly it is that we think we'll be on this earth for so long. Not that cancer is a death sentence, because it's not— but it is an eye-opener. It has made me realize that I need to make more of an effort to be present, enjoy the time that I have, and (as my end-of-treatment tattoo states) "Be still." We spend so much time making the big plans in life that sometimes we overlook the importance of the present moment. When worry inevitably creeps in—when I get a headache, when I have a scan scheduled, when a muscle feels sore one day—I remind myself to "be still." I'm here now, and that's what matters. That phrase comes from one of my favorite verses in the bible, Exodus 14:14: "The Lord will fight for you; you need only to be still."

By the end of the first day, 75 friends and family members had joined the group, and it kept growing from there. Whenever someone sent me a card or letter, I'd add them to the group. They had invested time to reach out to me, so it made sense to invite them inside this experience.

Sometime within the first week or two, my cousin called me to ask how things were going. She wasn't on Facebook, so she hadn't been hearing the latest updates. That's when my husband said, "Maybe you should start a blog, too." So I did: HoldingSpaceWithShelly.com. The blog and the Facebook page were essentially the same, though I limited photos of my girls to the Facebook page for privacy.

Prior to this, I wasn't a writer at all. When I first started writing updates, I was just sharing basic information and a lot of straightforward facts. But once treatment was underway and there weren't medical updates every day, I started to use the two platforms to share more personal thoughts about what was happening to me. The more I shared, the more I realized how therapeutic it was. Sometimes it helped me to better understand myself and to process everything as I had to put the thoughts and feelings into words.

Typically during chemo, I posted on the blog only when I felt like it. When I was partway through treatment, my friend at church said, "I can't believe how great you're doing." I was taken aback because, in fact, I was really struggling. All of the miserable chemo side effects had been in full force for several days leading up to that. I hadn't slept well for weeks. And I felt like I was failing as a mother because I was too tired to do a lot of things I would normally do.

"I'm not doing well at all—where'd you get that idea?" I asked her.

"I follow everything you post on Facebook and the blog," she answered, "and it sounds like you're doing really great."

That's when I realized that I was only posting on my good days and my best moments, often near the end of a chemo cycle. After all, who would want to take time to write after not sleeping all night, throwing up in the morning, and barely having enough energy to walk one block to get the girls on the bus? I would be down and depressed, sick and tired for a week. Then, as I was coming out of it, I'd feel better—and that's when I'd write something along the lines of "That was awful, but I'm doing so much better now" or "That was terrible, but at least one more is over." I wasn't writing in the really bad spaces (which were actually when I need the most prayers and support). When I realized that, I got the nudge to start writing more—to give people a more authentic sense of what this experience was really like.

In the worst times of chemo, I experienced almost every side effect possible. I lost 20 pounds and felt so weak. I had no appetite. I felt pain and discomfort in so many of my body systems. I had no hair and lost most of my fingernails and toenails. I had mouth sores that made talking painful, let alone trying to eat. So I survived on gas station slushies and Ensure. As I laid in the bathtub one night, after crying for three hours straight because of a particularly difficult bathroom issue, I perseverated on the thought that none of this made sense to me. I questioned what kind of world this is, with disease and suffering that seems so unnecessary.

At that point, I recognized my struggling faith. So I offered a prayer that would become routine for me through the hardest times, asking God to hold onto me, because I knew my grip to Him was letting loose. "Don't let me go," I prayed. He knew my heart, He knew my doubts and my limited comprehension. He knew how unfair I thought this was to my young daughters, to see their mom suffer and even have the potential of losing her. If He could just hold onto me while I struggled, I knew that when this was done I'd be able to reset my grip again. And I have.

This kind of faith struggle was hard for me to admit. But one day I wrote about it in the blog, and the response I got was so supportive. Other Christian friends affirmed that this didn't make me any less of a Christian. They would pray for my faith to hold strong. Hearing that they would pray for me through this was exactly what I needed. And this showed me the benefit of being vulnerable. Opening myself up to others allowed them to help in the ways that I needed most.

Other times, writing allowed me to move forward. For example, I kept the memory of my "diagnosis day" in my mind for a year. I didn't realize how much mental energy I was spending storing those details in my mind. But on the year anniversary of the diagnosis, I wrote all those details on my blog. And my mind suddenly felt lighter—more free. Finally I could let go of it and move on.

I was diagnosed on January 20th, 2017. Chemotherapy started February 9th and finished June 22nd. A little more than a month later, I had a bilateral mastectomy. Then I had radiation treatment, from October through November 2017. And the final major surgery was reconstruction in November 2018. As I write this, I still have one more step in the reconstruction process and then hopefully done forever!

Social media has provided a perfect platform for me to share information about my diagnosis and treatment. But it also provided a system to share another huge part of this experience for our family. I was cutting hours down at work, the medical bills were going to be piling up until I could pay off my out-of-pocket maximum, and expenses were being added to our budget (like parking at appointments, eating out more often, and those ridiculously expensive wigs). Looking at our finances, the first things that made sense to eliminate were extracurricular activities—our daughters' dance classes, cheerleading, and piano lessons—and canceling our previously planned trip to Disney.

One day at work, I opened up to one my closest friends, Aubree, about running out of "paid time off." My amazing co-workers had donated a lot of their time to me, but even that wasn't going to be enough to cover all of my absence. I was crying and told her, "I don't know how I'm going to tell the girls they have to stop taking dance classes. And we're going to have to cancel our Disney trip." She immediately said, "What if we do a GoFundMe page?" At first I said no, because I couldn't imagine taking money from people for these "extra" things. Vacation was a luxury we could postpone. Dance classes would be there next year when this was over.

But after a few more days, Aubree mentioned it again, and I hesitantly agreed to let her do it. We made a short video to introduce ourselves on the page and set a goal of $6,000. That goal was reached and exceeded within a few days! Support started pouring in—from friends we see frequently, long-time friends from our hometown just outside of Pittsburgh, friends from elementary school whom we had only recently connected with through Facebook. People came out of the woodwork to help our family. Every day we would get messages from people who had donated to help, and it was unreal. I cried every time I got another message from someone who helped us.

Within a few weeks, we exceeded our goal and raised over $15,000. The gratitude we feel for that financial support is hard to put into words. That money eliminated a huge source of stress during a time when everything else was challenging. It took away an enormous sense of guilt I had for missing work and bringing home smaller paychecks. But, more importantly in my mind, it allowed our girls to continue their fun activities in the evenings and maintain their routine. Instead of a year of no birthday parties, we were able to host parties outside our home, where we could show up and everything was taken care of. It even allowed Rob and me to take a special trip together to Lake Tahoe between chemo and surgery. And it allowed us not to spend all our savings, so we could still go to Disney World after everything was over. The trip was postponed but not canceled.

Another wonderful thing happened specifically to my girls during that very challenging time. That year, my daughters' principal nominated both of the them for the superintendent's annual "Courageous Kids" award. They were picked up at school by a limousine during the middle of the day and taken out to lunch with the superintendent and a handful of other students from the district. It was a surprise that they loved. They even received a special "VIP" nametag on a lanyard to wear, which they both held onto as a keepsake. They felt so special saying "We've ridden in a limo now, and Mommy and Daddy haven't even done that!" Those girls deserved it, too. All of it. They went through a year of hell with us, and they were more resilient and brave through it than I could've ever imagined. I'm so proud of them and hope resilience is ingrained in their character as they grow.

The GoFundMe and my daughters' recognition awards inspired me to try to raise money to help children of parents who are going through cancer treatment. A whole family goes through treatment, even if only one of them has the diagnosis. I want to help other families, so their children don't have to quit dance classes or skip birthday parties. We have a local nonprofit organization in Akron called Stewart's Caring Place that offers many activities to help people during cancer treatment. I'm currently working with their staff to figure out how to raise money specifically for children of survivors, because no one fights this alone.

I've also been inspired to continue with my writing. Many people commented that they enjoyed reading my writing and thought I should write a book. I didn't take it too seriously- most of them were family members, so of course they'd say that. But between their feedback and how much the writing was helping me, I figured I'd keep going. I also have two friends who are nurses at oncology centers, and they told me it really helps them to read stories from a patient's perspective. I haven't worked out the details yet, but I'm looking into different options for publishing my story. I may even listen to my family and write a book after all.

Cancer has been a rollercoaster, full of emotions about life and death that I never expected to have at an early age. But I've also seen love and support from family, friends, coworkers, and strangers that I'll never forget. Now I have an additional purpose in life: to help others going through it and to help their caregivers. And this reciprocity of love and caring is what life is all about.

It's Like the Death Star,
But Your Head Doesn't Explode

Name: Nichole Wouters

Town: Macomb, Michigan

Diagnosis: Adenocarcinoma lung cancer; stage 4

Age at diagnosis: 27

Age now: 30

When I was diagnosed with lung cancer, I was in the best shape of my life. I had a six pack. I was waking up at 3:45 in the morning to work out before I went to school, where I was a math teacher and varsity volleyball coach. I had started having trouble breathing, and I'd slept for 17 hours and missed Thanksgiving, and I was feeling sick and nauseous sometimes—but lung cancer? When the doctor said, "You have lung cancer," I was like, "You have the wrong person." It felt like an episode of *Grey's Anatomy* where they'd switched my chart with someone else's. Next thing I knew, they had put me on oxygen 24/7. I was 27 years old. My first question was, "Can we go to the casino with my oxygen tank? Because I feel like one of those old people."

When I was diagnosed, my doctor told me that lung cancer tends to metastasize to the bones or brain first. Nothing showed up on the PET scan for my bones. I got the brain scan done to make sure that looked OK. When I got the results, I was at my school putting in for leave. My phone rang, and it was my oncologist: "Hi, Nichole. I just needed to let you know that your brain scan is back and there's a spot, and we need to get that treated."

I almost blacked out at that point. Up until then, I was still thinking the whole thing was fake. Like they got the wrong biopsy report back. This "spot" was an 11 millimeter lesion over the motor strip of my brain. I would've lost control of my left side if it had grown another millimeter or two. I had no symptoms from it. After hearing this news, I lost it. That was when it all became real.

I was still on the phone with my doctor. She asked, "Is anyone with you?" I handed the phone to my sister and walked out. I was having tunnel

> BEST ADVICE: My sisters told me, "Who cares what everyone else thinks? They can shut the eff up and deal with it. Do what you want to do. Do what makes you happy." You don't think that you care what everybody thinks, but you do. And going through this, you're so self-conscious. But the best advice is: ignore everybody and do what makes you happy.

vision. I ran into my good friend, Claire, and grabbed her and started crying. I had already texted her about the cancer. Now I walked up to her, started crying, and whispered, "It's in my effing brain." I had no control over my emotions. She was strong for me.

The next day, I met with a radiation oncologist and we scheduled Gamma Knife radiation for a week later. But before they did that, they put me on an anti-seizure medication as a precaution, because of the location of the spot. I lost my memory on it—I just blanked. I ended up going to the hospital for a couple of days. My doctor thinks it may have been PTSD combined with the medication. I was released after the medication was out of my system, but the idea that I could lose my memory was scary.

Gamma Knife is targeted radiation, a higher dose all to one spot. The way they explained it to me, it's like the Death Star in *Star Wars*. All the lasers come together and then shoot. They added, "Except your head doesn't explode." It made me laugh.

After Gamma Knife I began chemo, with six treatments to start. Between my first CT scan before diagnosis and my first scan after I'd started chemo, the cancer seemed to have grown in my lungs. It was a scary idea that chemo wasn't making it better. I was feeling better—the scan just didn't show it. But the next scan was better. The chemo was working. After some time, the pathology came back, and I found out the cancer was HER2 positive. HER2 is typical for breast cancer but really rare for lung cancer. With lung cancers, 30% is small-cell and 70% is non-small-cell. There are three or four types of non-small-cell; adenocarcinoma is part of that. And then there are all these mutations in the cancer cells, and HER2 is like 2% of that. Just proof that no two cancers are the same.

I've had many different forms of treatment. My first type of chemotherapy was Carboplatin and Alimta. Once they found out about the HER2, I was put on a pill called Gilotrif. That was probably my best treatment if I had to pick one, because of mild side effects. I was on that for about six months; then it stopped working. I did Kadcyla and Nerlynx, a typical combination for breast cancer, for about four months. The Nerlynx was the worst. It was awful.

Scans showed that again I had progression, so I went back to Carboplatin and Alimta—but with immunotherapy, Keytruda, as well. I had been on a platinum chemo too, but I reached the maximum levels of it and they couldn't use it anymore. I didn't last long on the new combination and went on to try another immunotherapy. Once that didn't work, it was another combination of chemotherapies, Taxotere and Cyramza. Once I appeared stable, I was sent to Texas to participate in a T-cell therapy clinical trial. It was a similar process to a stem cell transplant. Unfortunately, the scans came back that it was unsuccessful, and I am now back to Taxotere and Cyramza.

I've had Gamma Knife radiation five times now, on 20 lesions in my brain. When you're getting Gamma Knife done, they screw a headpiece to your skull. During the second procedure, one of the screws hit a nerve on the back of my head and it was numb for about four months. I burnt my head with a blow-dryer because I didn't feel it getting hot. And then when I started getting feeling back, that nerve pain returned. Even brushing my hair with a really soft brush hurt. I'm happy, though, that Gamma Knife has been successful for me over the last few years. I hope that it continues to help in the future.

I was diagnosed in January of 2017. The volleyball season was over, so I didn't have to worry about my team at that time, even though I knew many were worried about me. I took off the spring, letting my body recover. And then I was back and feeling really good that August. I missed I think one tournament and one game, total, during my time of coaching with my cancer diagnosis (now two seasons). I just don't like sitting around. I hated sitting at home the whole time during chemo—hated it. I loved being around family, and it was nice to relax, but I was miserable. I was more depressed sitting at home. My goal had been to take a couple days off here and there, when needed, but I wasn't going to miss the school year.

Sometimes I worried that coaching and teaching while I was sick would hurt my students, even if it helped me. But for some of them, it was actually nice to see me and see that I could be working. They knew that I was going to keep living. They're great kids. This past year, I was in and out of the classroom for treatments all the time, but they kept doing things that needed to be done. Their level of maturity and understanding was amazing. They would email me when I was out and be like, "How are you? What's going on?" They wanted to know.

And they followed me on Twitter. Right after I was diagnosed, I was getting emails and messages from students, parents, coworkers, etc., asking, "What's going on? We heard rumors. We heard this." And I was just like, "OK, let's get this over with." I got on Twitter the night I was diagnosed. Overnight, I ended up having 900 followers. It blew up. I post random tweets with pictures on occasion, or small updates of my health. I have this really goofy habit of naming my medical equipment. My oxygen tank is called a Lincare, so I named it Linda. I posted a picture with the message, "Everybody meet Linda, my new best friend." My portable oxygen tank is called Phil. I try to keep the attitude light and positive. In recent months I made an Instagram account called "stickit2_cancer," where I blog my days and wear a different lipstick every day to make myself feel pretty. It's just little things that help me.

Because I'm already stage 4 and it's already metastasized, I will have to be on treatment all the time. If I take a break, it would be for quality of life. With these treatments, I can't get pregnant. It would kill me, the baby, or both. That was heartbreaking for me. I've come to terms with it, but it's hard. I make terribly inappropriate joke about it with my students. They would comment, "You're gonna do this to your own kids," and I'd say, "I can't have kids." They eventually began responding, "Well you can adopt me." They learned to deal with my humor and remember to keep life positive. I may not be a mother, but I am an aunt, and I love that. My niece was born this past November, and she is everything to me. I also have a fur baby, who I hope to train to be a therapy dog.

During the period of about eight months when I felt really good, I joined a volleyball league and was able to play for a while. I went on a couple of those adventure-type cancer-survivor trips and was super active. I went surfing and mountain biking. But after a while, being that active just made me tired. As my condition has worsened, I've had to make difficult choices about what I do and don't do. I decided to step down from coaching. It was a very difficult decision for me—it broke my heart. I told the players in person and cried. This was a passion of mine, and these girls and the community will forever be part of my family.

Missing out on things has been terrible. I'll walk up stairs now and have to sit down for like 10, 15 minutes because I can't breathe. I just end up coughing. Humidity and cold weather tend to make it worse. I just have to hope for the best. I've been on and off oxygen for the last two years. I ended up getting a portable concentrator, with two battery packs so it doesn't run out of air for about eight hours total. I still wear it when I sleep and when I'm active, but when I'm sitting around I hate wearing it, so I just don't. That's probably bad.

I have an amazing support system. I'm really, really, really, really lucky. My family is awesome. My sisters are my best friends. We're all two years apart. I spend all my time with my sisters and my parents. I'm happy with that, because they're my connection. Three of my sisters are nurses. My family comes to treatments with me. Sometimes, there are seven people there with me. My parents help me out at home with getting around. My dad comes to all of the treatments, no matter what.

When I was diagnosed, I was single, and I used to joke, "Are there cancer dating apps?" I was living with my parents. I was going through all of this. I'm like, "None of this is sexy." Like, "Hey, you can't breathe." Or "I don't want to go out with oxygen tubes." I came to the conclusion, "I'm never going to meet anyone. That's fine. Whatever."

Before I was diagnosed, my best friend's husband sent me a text about a guy he knew. I had just ended things with another guy and wanted to be single for a while. Over the next few months, he kept bringing this guy up, but then I was diagnosed and I didn't want to deal with it. Last summer he brought him up again, and I was like, "All right, just give the guy my number. I'll get rid of him. I'll scare him off." But he was persistent and sarcastic and funny and caring. He would text me every day like, "Hey, how are you?" He had correct grammar, and I was just like, "Who is this?" Eventually he asked, "Can we go on a date? Can I meet you?"

Our first date we went to a brewery and had dinner, then went to a comedy show. It was just so original and fun, and we laughed. It felt weird to be happy. At the time I was on a pill treatment, so I felt very normal. It was hard to make him realize that things wouldn't always be that stable. We kept dating. I was coaching volleyball. He would come to the volleyball tourna-ments and watch my team. He just wanted to spend time with me. He knew about the cancer before we even started dating. He knew it had metastasized. He knew all of this, and he still wanted to be with me.

He was amazingly supportive. Nerlynx created awful stomach issues, including diarrhea. My third date, I was saying, "I need to go to CVS," because I didn't have Immodium on me. And he's like, "What? What's going on?" I told him about the side effects, and he said, "Oh, did I tell you about the time that I crapped my pants on the side of the road?" He made everything OK and humanized what I was going through.

Another example: Thanks again to Nerlynx, I shit the bed while we were in Vegas staying with one of my friends. I woke up and started crying hysterically because I did this in bed next to him. He was like, "It's fine. You're OK. We'll put everything in the washing machine."

Unfortunately life and relationships take many turns, and we ended up going our separate ways. I wish him nothing but the best. The relationship helped me to realize that I'm still beautiful and worth someone's love.

One of my ways of coping when I'm afraid is to crack jokes. Not good ones, either, and normally pretty dark. When I'm facing something scary, I make fun of it until it's there and it's real. I'm still in denial half the time about my situation. I just keep moving—I face it head on. I'm afraid of spiders, OK, but I refuse to be afraid of my treatments. I'm not afraid of surgeries. At first I didn't lose my hair. Once I did start losing my hair, I took the situation into my own hands and shaved it—in front of 600 high school 9th-graders, the varsity football team, and the marching band. I just wanted to show the students that even when you're afraid of what's happening, you can take control.

What I'm realizing now, and what I wish I'd known at the beginning, is that the unknown doesn't always need to be scary. Yes, there are days when I lay in bed, don't want to do anything, and get upset. It's OK to have those emotions, but it's not OK to let them cripple you. I spent a lot of time being scared and a lot of time just thinking, *This is the end. This is it.* And it was never it. Just keep going—*that's it.*

SOUTHEAST

The World's First Farewell to the Rectum Party

. . . .

Name: Pat Bodenhamer

Town: Paragould, Arkansas

Diagnosis: Colorectal cancer

Age at diagnosis: 38

Age now: 46

I am an Ordained Elder in the United Methodist Church. At the time of my diagnosis, I was serving two small churches in North Arkansas, in Diamond City and Omaha. I had been their pastor for about three years. Both churches were mostly elderly people in their retirement. We were having a great time loving God together. I was single and living alone. My mom, my dad, and all my relatives all lived in Mountain Home, Arkansas, about an hour away.

Things started when I felt bad for about two weeks—just run down. One day I was at church working in the food pantry, and when I used the restroom, there was blood in my stool. I called my Dad, who is a retired ER nurse. He said, "Patty, it's probably nothing major. You probably just have hemorrhoids. Women your age get hemorrhoids. Or you could just be all stopped up. Go to the ER. I'll call them and tell them you're coming." He was out of town at the time.

WORST ADVICE: When an acquaintance found out that I chose to stay at Mountain Home to get my treatment, she called and said, "You are going to die if you do not come to University of Arkansas Medical School." And I said, "Whoa, sister. This is the best choice for me and my family." So I would say the worst advice is when someone says, "This is the only place that can heal you." There are many different places. You have to find what works for you and where you feel comfortable.

Mountain Home, my hometown, is a small community. My Dad spent 38 years working in the ER there, so everybody at the hospital had watched me grow up. I went to the emergency room, and they did an X-ray. They said, "Yeah, you're a little backed up. We're going to give you something to clean you out. Don't worry about it." Then they sent me home.

That was on February 13th of 2012. I took all the nasty stuff—but only felt worse and worse. My mom came over and stayed with me. On Friday morning I said, "Mom, something's wrong." We called my dad, who was still out of town. He said, "Go back to the ER. They're probably going to do a rectal exam, so prepare yourself."

We went, and they did a rectal. They felt the tumor—and it was like whoever had watched me grow up in that hospital came alive and rushed down to the emergency room. They got my dad, who was on his way home, on his cell phone. They called Dr. Stahl, a surgeon who knew me. He was in surgery but said on speakerphone, "Patty, I'll be right down. I gotta close this lady up." I said, "Please take care of her first!"

It was a flurry of activity. By that time it was late in the afternoon, almost closing time, but they decided to do my colonoscopy anyway. It is not typical that doctors will stay around on a Friday afternoon, but the doctor was one whose kids I used to babysit, and he stayed.

I was so dehydrated that they couldn't get an IV started. They said, "We can do it without drugs," and I said, "Do it. Let's go." They wheeled me back, wide awake. I saw the tumor myself on the screen.

"It looks really bad," I said.

"It is," the doctor answered. "Are you ready to fight?"

"Let's do it."

It was a fairly large mass. It was impeding my colon so much that nothing was passing through. They said it may have been growing in there for years but had finally dropped down and started causing problems.

My dad arrived. My mom was there with me. My dad immediately went to talk to the doctor. When he came back, he crawled in bed with me. He said, "It's cancer." And we cried. That was a Friday. Somebody called the Bishop, and he was going to send someone to fill in for me. I overheard the conversation and said, "No, they're mine." I had worked hard on a really great sermon for Sunday, and I wanted to preach it. I told the leadership, "Please don't tell anybody. This is important for me. I want to tell my churches."

That Sunday, my family and my best friends all come to church. Congregants were thinking, *Why is everybody here? Pat must be getting moved to another church.* I preached this great sermon. God is just so amazing. The sermon I had prepared was about the idea that God opens new gates for us, but we have to close the old ones to go through. At the end I said, "God closed a gate for me, and he's opened another one—one that I don't have any choice but to go through."

I told them that I had colorectal cancer. They were so supportive. The Bishop offered to put me on disability and send a new pastor. They said, "No, she's ours. We will take care of her." I was out of the pulpit for an entire year, and they paid my salary and took such good care of me. They remodeled my parsonage while I was gone. They were just wonderful.

My parents are divorced. My dad had married my stepmother, Kathy, and she is an RN too. Even though I grew up living with my mom, I decided to stay with Dad and Kathy because they could take care of me if anything happened. It was the best decision. Growing up, my dad was both there and not there. Now he became my coach and my cheerleader. One gift of everything happening was that we would grow to be very close.

The next week, I met my oncologist and we put a treatment plan together. Sometime that week, I decided to visit the cemetery. When my great grandma was alive, she ran the cemetery, so it's a special place to me. My Dad called while I was on my way, but I told him I was going to my mother's. He said, "Well, OK. Where are you right now?" I said, "I'm just on the road, Dad." I was almost at the cemetery, and he said, "Now where are you?" I said, "I'm just going to Mom's, Dad." He said, "Well, I'm at the cemetery, and I'm right behind you." He told me he had wanted to sit with our relatives, to think and pray. So we sat there together. I said, "If this thing goes bad, I'm OK to die. I know where I'm going, and it's OK."

Within two weeks of getting my diagnosis, I started radiation. They wanted to shrink the tumor before surgery, so I did six months of radiation and 24-hours-a-day, seven-days-a-week chemo, through a port placed in my arm. I've never been a real modest person, but during radiation, any modesty I did have got pitched out the door. You're laying there with your rear end up in the air. The nurses always tried to keep me covered, but I said, "Ladies, it's cool. I really don't care. Just do what you gotta do." I said to myself, *If you don't laugh, you're gonna cry all through this thing.* I remember one day the radiation students came through. I couldn't see them, just their feet, but I said, "Take a picture, kids. It's a Kodak moment."

Every day, my dad took me to radiation and then back home. Three or four weeks after I started, the side effects hit me hard. I only got sick a couple of times, but I was so tired. I would get in the door and have to lie down in the kitchen and nap, right there. Most days I slept all day. My dad was the medical person, and my stepmother helped me with baths and that sort of thing. My mom was working, and she would come out overnight and take me to movies or on walks, to get me out of the house.

What helped the most during some of that time was all the cards and notes people sent, since I couldn't have visitors. I have a box full of them, some of them from people I didn't even know who had heard about me from their preachers. They're from all over. It was so powerful to me that someone would take the time to write me a note.

The majority of my cancer battle was fought with a positive attitude and the knowledge that God was walking with me every step of the way. But I also knew I needed time to cry, to be angry, to yell. So I set my phone timer and gave myself 30 minutes a day. During that 30 minutes I could cuss at God, be mad, and say whatever I wanted. So many times people feel guilty for being mad at God. But God's big enough to take that.

During hard moments, I adopted a saying that I still use today: *I rest in the arms of Jesus, and I lean on the prayers of many.* Every PET scan, I said that over and over as my mantra. I rest in the arms of Jesus. I lean on the prayers of many. I knew that so many people were praying for me. And I knew that healing comes in many different forms. Sometimes healing is death. So I wanted to rest in Jesus, knowing that whatever his healing was, it was gonna be OK.

The mantra really helped me, but I had my mini breakdowns, too. Early on, when it got to be too much, I told my dad, "I need some happy drugs here." My dad said, "Let's go see Dr. Bufford." He was an ER doctor my dad had worked with. We went out to his house, where he was working cattle. Remember—we're in rural Arkansas. He wanted to be a vet and ended up being a people doctor. I told him, "Man, Doc, I just need something to take the edge off." I was falling into depression, and I knew it was not going to help in the healing process. He reassured me and said, "It is OK for you not to be strong all the time." That was very powerful to me. I said to myself, OK, I will take my drugs, and I will not be ashamed.

I did my six months of chemo and radiation. I was so burnt on the inside from the radiation that afterward, I took a month off to heal. Then we scheduled surgery. During one of the consultations, Dr. Stahl brought his colostomy nurse in, and they started talking about placement. I said, "Whoa, what are you doing?" And he said, "Well, you're going to have a permanent colostomy." I hadn't realized it until that moment. All my positive thinking just left the room. It was rough. All I can remember is going home and crying uncontrollably.

The next morning I woke up and said, "Well, I can be pissed off, or I can be happy that I've been given a second chance."

We scheduled the surgery for May 20th. At that point I said to myself, "Well, how are we going to say goodbye to my rectum?" I decided to throw a Farewell to the Rectum party. Why not? Of course, we had it at a Mexican restaurant, with whoopee cushions as party favors and those cream-filled horns as colons. I invited some of my closest friends and family. They all said, "We've never been to a Farewell to a Rectum party," and I said, "I've never had one." There's a first time for everything!

We had one hell of a party. People in the restaurant were laughing. It was a great hangover the next morning, but it was so worth it. My sister picked up my liquor bill, and she went, "Dang, Patty."

I decided to name my colostomy. I named it Ray, after Dr. Stahl. The news went through the hospital, and everybody was talking about Ray the Colostomy. When May 20th arrived, I told my mom, "I want to go to the bathroom one more time. I just want to say goodbye to my rectum." So I went to the bathroom, at Baxter Regional in Mountain Home, and I said, "Uh, thank you for serving me well for 38 years. I'm sorry you had to turn on me, and now you have to come out."

It's a hard surgery. They cut you from end to end. I ended up in ICU. What was supposed to be a two- to three-day stay in the hospital turned out to be 20 days. I did not bounce back at all. I had lots of problems and was getting weaker and weaker. Finally they decided to put a picc line in and give me sustenance through IV and blood transfusions.

At one point I had broken one of the stitches loose in my stoma, so Dr. Stahl performed a little surgery right there in my hospital bed, with what seemed like 30 people from the ER, including my dad, gathered around watching. They were having a big reunion. I thought, Well, I'm so glad that my body can provide all this fun.

The first time they got me up to walk, the pain was horrible. We ended up wrapping a sheet around my midsection like a tourniquet. It took five people to get me up, every time. Two days before my release, I found out that the Relay for Life, an annual event that raises money for cancer research, celebrates survivors, and remembers those who lost their battles, was happening. I told my dad I was going. He said, "Now, Patty, you've had a rough go." I said, "No, I'm taking my lap. I'm going."

I was released the day of the race. We took a wheelchair, and my mom and dad and stepmom and other supporters walked me around that survivor's lap.

Recovery was hard. My stepmom, God love her, she cleaned me up every day and taught me how to change my colostomy. Talking about it makes me emotional. Then I started another three months of chemo. Again, I didn't lose my hair, but I developed neuropathy in my hands, feet, and mouth. I couldn't touch anything cold; when I drank water, it had to be warm. I would get lockjaw, which was probably the roughest part besides the surgery recovery. I still suffer from the neuropathy in my hands and my feet, and in my tongue and lips when I'm really tired. I also gained over 100 pounds. But, you know, I was alive. I just had to laugh it off.

On February 14th of 2013, I was going to have my first PET scan since I'd finished chemo. I told my mom, "We're having a party." We planned this huge party at the church, "Kicking the Hell Out of Cancer," for the next day, when we'd get the results. We decorated with balloons. We had over 400 people RSVP from all over the state.

Everybody at the hospital was concerned, saying, "What if the results are that the cancer's back?" That day, we took a break from decorating for the party to get the results. My Dad said, "OK, what if this turns out badly?" And I said, "Then we'll make it a kick-off party to the next." We'd have the party, whatever the result.

So we got the results, then we went down and had our party. At first we didn't tell anyone. I waited until everyone was together and celebrating, then made the announcement: "We got the all-clear!" Everyone jumped up and cheered. Many broke out in tears. I remember standing in front of all those people, realizing, if this had gone the other way, these people would still be here, cheering me on and supporting my family.

Every Relay for Life, I take my lap and cry the entire time. This past year, I hit my five-year-clean mark. Of course, I had a party. My doctors came, and we had a great time.

Throughout my cancer journey, I made a point of being very open and honest about what was happening to me. Since nobody ever talks about it, I had no idea what to expect when I was going through it. I wanted to take that shame away. I didn't cause this. I didn't ask for cancer. After my treatment, I spoke to an 8th-grade graduating class. I told them, "Be who you are, and don't be ashamed of that." At the end of it, I revealed that I was a "bag lady." I got these really weird looks, like, "What do you mean, you're a bag lady?" I pulled out one of my colostomy bags, and I explained what it was. I said, "Even being a 'bag lady,' I could make a difference. And you can make a difference in your life."

Our church leadership, the Bishop and district superintendents, don't know what to do with clergy who have cancer. We don't want to be removed from our calling. We want to live out our calling through our cancer. Around 12 clergy people from all over the country have called me and said, "I just got this diagnosis." So I've walked with them, and been with them during surgeries. Some of the churches that I've served, I call it "the club that nobody wants to be in." About two weeks ago, I received a call from a pastor who said, "I think I need my invitation." I always send them a box of goodies that they'll need for chemo and radiation. Socks, a teddy bear, and other things that helped me get through it. I call it the "They Messed with the Wrong Person Box." I decorate it.

Just this week, one of my church members learned he has to have a colostomy. I went to him, pulled down the front of my pants, and said, "Let me introduce you to Ray. He's not very pretty. He's very annoying, and he stinks sometimes. But this is what keeps me alive."

Not too long ago, I was working on a sermon called "Dear Younger Me." During my diagnosis and treatment, I had moments when I thought that I was less of a woman because I had cancer and a colostomy. The sermon became my chance to tell my younger self, "You are a beautiful woman of God, and not even cancer can take that away." I know now I came out of the experience a better person. Fewer body parts, but a better person—one who can face whatever comes my way.

Lighting a Fire with Reading

Name: Andrea Liliana Griffiths

Town: Bradenton, Florida

Diagnosis: Breast cancer; stage 3; invasive lobular carcinoma

Age at diagnosis: 35

Age now: 37

I can remember the moment of my diagnosis so clearly, sitting in front of the doctor with my husband and listening to her say, "Unfortunately I don't have good news. It's an invasive lobular carcinoma." It was the worst news I'd ever had in my life, but I was still hopeful. My mother had beaten breast cancer when I was a child. *This is gonna be a horrible year, but we'll make it*, I thought. *Whatever it is, we'll take it on. Look at Baby Gladys!*

That's my mom's name. I call her "baby" to annoy her. When she was diagnosed, they gave her zero chance of making it, but she did. The reason I'm here in America to begin with is my mother's cancer.

Since I was diagnosed, she has been a lot more open with her story. She used to not talk about it at all, because it was a very sad time in her life. I was 10 and my brother was 7 when she left our home in Cali, Colombia, as a last measure to save her life. In Colombia, there were only so many re-

BEST ADVICE: Quit wasting your time thinking about *what if, what if.* Just be right now: *Right now I'm OK, right now I'm fine.* Worrying was my thing. I wish I'd spent less time thinking about the worst possible outcomes and been more focused on believing in a good one.

sources at the hospital where she was being seen. Her doctor told her, "You're very young. You have small children. If you really want a fighting chance, try to find your way to America.'

So she did. Her story, her struggle, is amazing. She moved here as an illegal immigrant. She paid a coyote to take her through Mexico. She was treated in Houston. A friend she had in New York came there to care for her during chemotherapy. This country saved her life. When my mother went into remission, she moved to New York, fully intending to come back to Colombia—but by that time, there wasn't a home for her to come back to. About a month after she left Colombia, my father introduced my brother and me to our "new mom." He didn't wait any time to move on. So Mom decided to stay in New York and find a way to get us here. It finally happened when I was 17 and my brother was 14. She had married a U.S. citizen—but had to wait six years before she could leave to travel to Colombia, since she had come here illegally. At that point, she came for us and took us straight to the embassy to start the process of our becoming residents. We were blessed that we were able to do it.

When I called my mom to give her the news I had cancer, I didn't even know how to tell her. "I don't really have really good news," I said. Her reaction was very much like mine. "Remember how they told me to go to hospice, I wasn't going to make it? And look, I'm here so many years later. Now you're here, in the United States, and the technology's advanced so much." She was very positive—but also devastated, because of course she's a typical Latina mom. She cried like it was the end of the world, saying, "I can't believe this is happening to you, happening to me." It felt like history repeating itself.

Of course, I was terrified. My children were so young. My baby was just 1, and my son was 4. I just kept thinking, *How am I going to do this?* Every time I looked at my children I wanted to cry, thinking, *Oh my God, I can't be sick. How am I gonna be sick? They depend on me.* I did a lot of crying when I was in the shower. You try to keep a brave face for everybody, but at the same time you're like, Holy shit, am I really gonna make it?

I met with the oncologist right away, and a week later I had a chemo port in. I've had excellent, proactive care at a good VA hospital. I'm fortunate—I was injured while in the Army, just enough to qualify. (I enlisted when I was young and stupid, at 17, because I felt like I needed to give back to the country that had saved my mother. Wonderful experience—but I wouldn't recommend it.) My husband got permission from his employer to work at home, so he could help me with the boys. I really made it a point to try my hardest to not be sick in front of them. I'm curious to see what they remember of this time when they're older.

We were living right outside Orlando by Disney, so we had annual passes. I used to have my chemo rounds on either Monday or Tuesday, depending on my blood counts. I'd make it a point to think, OK, I know this week is gonna be awful, but by Saturday I'll be ready for Disney. It was always my goal to make it to Disney. It was the middle of the summer, super hot, but I felt like if I got out there with them and we were doing something that had nothing to do with me being bald and sick, everything would be OK. It wouldn't matter so much if there were days during the week where I was too sick to play. I'm like a 5-year-old myself, thinking Disney makes everything all right! We had the fast pass and would go for two or three hours a visit. We almost always made it.

When I shaved my head, I was terrified the baby wouldn't recognize me and my older son would be scared. None of that happened. It worked out fine. Mami was just bald, and sometimes Mami put on a wig, and sometimes she didn't. It didn't bother them at all.

When I had surgery, a double mastectomy, I was worried for my 4-year-old, because that's a huge change, and for the baby, because we couldn't cosleep anymore. And then you come home and you have these drains. I had four, which I tried my best to disguise. We're a very affectionate, in-your-face family, and I couldn't pick them up and do the physical things I usually do, like hugs before bed. I was lucky my in-laws came in, and they were able to look after them and distract them. My husband took care of the drains for me. We would go into our bedroom and close the door and tell the boys, "OK, mommy's having her operation." That's what we called it.

My husband always jokes with me, "You're like the nakedest person." And we've always been like that. It's like, it's my body, it's your body, it's nothing weird. After surgery, for the first time with my son, I thought, *Oh, I'm not sure I want him to see me like this*. But one day we didn't lock the bathroom door when my husband was helping me have a French bath, just a little spot-clean. He was helping me get dressed when my son popped in. My in-laws outside the room were freaking out—"Oh, don't go in there!" But all I did was look at him; and he just looked at me, and went on to tell us whatever he came to tell say, and then left. And that was that. We were all in a panic—"Oh my God, will be he scarred for life? Am I messing him up? Is he gonna remember this?" And honestly, he just came in and didn't even comment on what he saw. That was that. They're so much more resilient than we give them credit for.

I finished radiation in February 2018. I've been working since the end of chemo, throughout surgery and radiation. I interviewed for my job in a wig and sat through my last two rounds of chemo with my computer, working. Once I was on a call in my chemo chair, and my nurses were looking at me like, "She's a crazy person." But at that point, working helped me because it gave my brain something new to think about.

I'm confident that the surgeon got everything out. I really hope so. I haven't had a PET scan since surgery, and I really haven't had any post tests. My oncologist says I'm never "cured" and will always have to be more conscious. But to keep the fear managed, it's helping me to think of myself as in remission. I've had one more surgery, to start to prep for reconstruction, and later this year will have a full hysterectomy.

Once you hear that you have cancer, everything changes. The day I found out, we had already thought it was the "worst day ever"—that same day, my husband got news that he didn't get the job he had spent months interviewing for, a job that would have been life-changing for our family. Our perspective shifted very quickly. Cancer's like a giant Boogey Man, and now that I've seen him, I have to live with him. In the months since, we have had hard days and we have had good days. We have had disappointments and other health difficulties. We found out my 2-year-old is allergic to fish only after he had a terrible allergic reaction where we thought he was going to die. But things that would spin me into panic before don't do the same for me now. If anything happens with my husband, or we have any kind of disappointment at work, I tell him, "If that's the worst thing that happens to us today, we'll be just fine." Or if we're traveling and our flight is delayed, I say, "If this is the worst thing that happens on this trip…." I tend to look at things with a lot more perspective.

I am much more cheerful and grateful in my life overall. I find beauty in things I never noticed before. Chemo became a time to reconnect with some of the things I used to enjoy but had stopped doing when I became a parent. With parenting, your focus completely shifts, and you go weeks where you're *getting by, getting by, getting by.* Your time is not your own anymore, or at least that was the way I was looking at it. I used to read a lot. So during chemo I started reading again for pleasure. I read *One Hundred Years of Solitude* and *Love in the Time of Cholera* again—books that were huge for me as a Colombian growing up. I found a lot of comfort in them, because they reminded me of when life was simpler.

Just after I finished radiation, I woke up one morning and happened to see a Tweet that it was Gabriel Garcia Marquez' birthday. Normally I would remember this day myself, because he was such a big author in my life. Colombians are very proud of their culture and country. Usually we make the news for horrible things, like drug cartels and kidnappings. Marquez is our one export that everybody loves. The entire world adores him. When I saw that Tweet, it reminded me so much of my childhood and an earlier version of myself.

I had already been thinking that I wanted to write about memory and how the brain works. My brain has not been the same since I had chemo. I honestly believe, even though my oncologist says this is a myth, that chemo brain is a real thing. I was a lot sharper before than I am now. Now I need to make a conscious effort to do things that before came very naturally. And yet my senses will surprise me with these powerful memories of childhood. Like when it's really warm and it rains, that smell of the rain hitting the concrete takes me back. So I wanted to write something about that. When I saw the Tweet about Marquez' birthday, I thought, *Oh my God, it's today. Let's do it today.*

I published the essay I wrote on Medium, and it closes this way: "Gabo said it best: 'It is not what happens to you, but what you remember and how you remember it.'" From the past year, I'll choose to remember the love I felt from friends old and new, the generosity of my colleagues, the compassion of my husband, and the happiness in my children's eyes when I got home from the hospital. I've learned a lot. My battle is not over, but for right this moment the battlefield is calm. My hair is growing, my energy is coming back, and I'm reading again, lighting a fire in myself to write and to share. If I can share one lesson with you today, it'll be more a request: to take a second to find the pleasant smell and the beautiful colors, to engrave them in your heart and ask your brain to remember the good parts. We are all dying, after all—just not yet, and hopefully for me not for at least another 63 years.

The Alchemist,
Transforming Fear into Love
· ·

Name: Maimah Karmo

Town: Aldie, Virginia

Diagnoses: Breast cancer; stage 2; ER-, PR-, HER2- ("triple negative")

Age at diagnosis: 32

Age now: 44

I came to the United States from Liberia as a refugee when I was 15 years old. It took me a while to settle into life here—being displaced and losing everything I knew was a shock. But I knew that I'd make the best of my life. I always had a drive to succeed, so that was never in doubt. It took my family a few years to find our groove. Our main focus was on each person contributing, supporting each other, giving back to the community and church. We all worked and chipped in to support the household. At some point, I saved enough to go to college. Then I got into the workforce, and I grew in my career. I was focused on achieving the American dream. But there was something missing. I had been praying for a long time, asking God to show me my path. I had an intention to figure out how I could make a difference in this world.

Many years later, my life had changed in so many wonderful ways. I'd had a beautiful baby girl. In 2006, my daughter was 3 years old. I had just bought my first house and was living comfortably, thinking, *Finally, I can take a deep breath.* Then, taking a shower one morning, I found a lump in my breast. I knew that it didn't belong there, and I didn't have a good feeling. I felt panic well up inside me. If it was cancer, I could die and leave my daughter without a mother.

After I felt the lump, the doctor sent me for a mammogram. It didn't show anything, because my breasts are dense. My OBGYN then referred me to a breast surgeon, who performed an unsuccessful aspiration. He told me, "You're too young. Come back in six months to a year." Instead, I kept pushing the doctor and made her give me a biopsy a few months later. The next day, she called to tell me I had breast cancer. If I had listened to her initial advice, I might be dead today. The breast cancer I had was aggressive and triple negative—there's still no targeted treatment for this pathology. After diagnosis, I was in shock for months. I had surgery. I began chemotherapy in a deep, dark space. I was frightened and overwhelmed. I had surrendered all my power to the disease and the depression that I was feeling.

A couple of weeks into my second round of chemo, I was in the cancer shit—so frickin' scared I couldn't think straight. One of my friends said to me, "You're more powerful than this. What are you going to do with it? How are you going to use what's happened for something bigger than you?" And I was like, "I don't know. I don't understand any of this."

She wouldn't let me off the hook. "You have the power to change the world," she said. "This can be the way." At first I was really angry with her. I wanted her to leave me alone. But I didn't stop thinking about what she had said. She planted a seed for me that was really powerful. That day was a tough one for me. I was so angry at God. One night, spent, before I went to bed, I prayed that God would change my energy and attitude, and give me strength. I prayed that God would shift the way I was thinking and show me my purpose, and I promised that if He did, I would give my life back in service to others...and I woke up the next morning a new person.

That's when I had my big shift. I woke up to the fact that life doesn't promise anything to anybody. You can get in the car one minute to go run errands and not come back alive. You can go to bed and not wake up. It's all random, and no one lives forever. No longer could I be lulled into thinking that because I'm young, nothing will happen to me. It occurred to me that I had wasted so much time in my 32 years, chasing money and building a career and looking to get the house, the man, the dog, the 2.5 kids, and then someday retire. What cancer gave me was a gift of knowing that I have a finite amount of time, and to really focus on how I will use that time. I realized that I had a desire to make a difference in the world.

That's how I began my work. As my hair was falling out, I started to build the Tigerlily Foundation. The name was inspired by the beautiful stargazer lily and how, like a woman, it is beautiful and strong, transforming through the seasons of its life. Tigerlily was created with two things in mind. First, I wanted to ensure that no young woman goes through what I did—in terms of almost not finding the cancer, and feeling so lost and alone. I have an amazing mom who taught me to do my breast exams at 13. A lot of mothers may not be talking with their daughters about their breast health and knowing their body. So that was something I wanted to bring to the forefront of people's minds. I wanted young women to have the tools to be their own best advocate—and to speak up if a doctor's advice doesn't sit right.

Second, I wanted to give women a space to be authentic about what they are feeling, when they are feeling it, and how they are feeling it. I wanted to help them deal with those emotions and the life changes that come with breast cancer. When it came to support organizations, all I saw was *pink this* and *pink that* and walks and runs. Nobody was talking about the anxiety and the depression and the utter fear of something in your body trying to kill you. People just want to see you get better and say you're fine. But I wasn't fine. I wasn't fine during my treatment. I wasn't fine for a long time after. There was no space for me to give voice to the negative, but real, emotions. I wanted other women who look like me to see themselves in my story and become advocates for themselves. I wanted to give women a different way of seeing cancer—to see that even in this dark space, you can transform your life by becoming more intentional. You can wake up and live on purpose.

So that's how the organization evolved. At first, telling my story was very scary. Speaking with authority on anything medical, even from the patient's perspective, is scary. When I was asked to speak at events, doctors' attitudes seemed to be, "Well, you're not a doctor." Still, I kept at it. I was asked to go to Capitol Hill to share my story and help inform health policy. I started speaking on the news. Over time, I began to see the power of one person's voice, not just to change health care, but to inspire other survivors to see their power as well. The more comfortable I became in that space, the more I enjoyed it and believed I could really make a difference. I realized I was telling so much more than my own story—I was giving other girls and young women the permission to tell theirs, create change, and save lives. And then I wrote a book.

I love to create light. That's a life theme for me: replacing darkness with light. There's so much darkness around certain topics. Sometimes patients are depressed, anxious, or suicidal because they're so freaking scared. Some women's partners leave them after diagnosis, so the patient is left to deal with that plus her cancer journey. Or when treatment ends, and there is no plan for survivorship. Or caregivers, spouses, and children are trying to cope with their loved one's cancer journey or death. There is so little conversation around these issues, but they're real. I want to shine the light on things that people don't want to see. The more you give things light, the more you can improve them, and heal and empower people.

BEST ADVICE: One day when my daughter was about 6, I was washing dishes, agonizing about whether I was doing the right things with Tigerlily. Could I really blend my spiritual practices with helping young women and their families? In that moment of doubt, my daughter came up behind me and said, "Hey, Momma."

"What?"

"Do you believe?"

"What?"

"Do you *believe?*"

It was almost supernatural—a huge sign for me that, yes, I do believe, and I really have the power to inspire great change and make an impact on millions of lives, so I will.

Tigerlily Foundation is the way I channel all that light toward breast cancer survivors, patients, caregivers, and children—anyone affected by this disease. My days are full and passion-filled. I do my podcast, videos, blogs, and social media. I plan events and create ideas around how to serve this unique population in deeply authentic ways. And then I work with my team to create programming for patients, pursue funding, have meetings, and build partnerships.

My daughter is now 16 years old. I never hid things from her. She's very much a part of everything I've done. I took her to conferences and speaking engagements. When I had my first book signing, I would sign each book, and then she would sign too. She could see how I was changing and growing, and the impact of the work. And she saw me both happy and sad. She came to understand that you have to work on yourself first. As you evolve, your work evolves, and your desire to impact more people. As she grew, my daughter wanted to help people, so she launched an annual event called Pajama Glam that is quickly becoming one of our signature programs. It's a forum where girls and mothers can talk about breast health in a fun and open way. The event has really grown, and we are looking at doing it in other states. I'm really proud of her, and many of her friends are getting involved. It's exciting to see the next generation becoming empowered, becoming part of the solution.

Marian Wright Edelman said, "Service is the rent we pay for living." That's a quote I live by. People take their life for granted; we take our breath for granted. My soul's renting my body. And so the rent I pay for that is serving others, as a thankful gesture to God for allowing me the space to express myself on this planet at this time. Legacy starts when you're alive. It's not about waiting to die to make a difference or having an epitaph. What are you doing as you're alive to make the world a better place, right now, for those who are living in it?

For a long time, I was consumed by fear. Even when you are declared cancer-free, there is still that fear of it returning. I couldn't just go and "live my life" as the doctors had told me. I began reading all I could about diet, nutrition, mind-body connection, other healing modalities, food as medicine, yoga, breathing, energy work, and more. Even as the years passed after my diagnosis, I still sometimes feel the fear bubbling up. It's a choking, overwhelming uncertainty. But I think to myself: At the end of my life, when I measure my buckets of time, how many buckets will be given to the fear? How is it helping me? Since it's not, I know I need to find ways to transmute that energy into something positive. I need to transmute this cancer madness into magic, and I do that with passion and love. Fear has no place in love. So when I feel afraid, I find something to pour love and thankfulness into. That gets me through it. I have no control over when I leave this planet, but I can control what I do when I'm here.

I tell the patients I work with all the time that they need to feel what they feel. But after a while, I always come back to them with the same questions: Why are you here? What did you come for? What is your purpose? What do you want to do with this life? Working with them as they answer those questions, I see them transform before my eyes. This is so very powerful.

Why Save Me?
& Other Questions for God

Name: Rosalinda Macias

Town: Chesapeake, Virginia

Diagnosis: Acute lymphocytic leukemia; pre-b cell

Age at diagnosis: 17

Age now: 23

Leading up to my diagnosis, the symptoms were there. But it was junior year of high school, the year that everyone stresses is so important for college admissions. *Who participates in the most extracurricular activities? Who has the better grades? Who is president of this? Captain of that? Who is applying to the highest-tier colleges?* I had an incredible amount of fatigue and joint pain, but I figured it was all stress-related.

Attending mass together has always been a beloved tradition in my family. Those last couple of months before my official diagnosis, it became a burden to get ready. I dreaded going. I was in pain, my fatigue levels had increased, and I would go in sweatpants with a messy bun. Honestly, I looked like shit. I was too tired to do anything, but it still never occurred to me something might actually be wrong.

BEST ADVICE: I cannot stress this enough: Speak up for yourself! No one can advocate for yourself better than you. Speak up when you are concerned about anything. Don't stay silent. You are your best advocate. If you don't advocate for yourself, who will?

Everything took a turn for the worse on a family trip to West Virginia. My dad sells wholesale restaurant supplies and dinnerware. We drove up to Homer Laughlin's tent sale so we could source some inventory. The drive was horrible (for me at least), because my joint pain jumped from a 3 to a 4 to a 10. I had never in my life experienced pain like that. I complained the entire drive there. It had to have been the longest 7 hours of my life. Of course, Father Dearest thought it was my way to get out of working (spoiler alert: It wasn't).

That night in the hotel, I developed a fever. I also got my period. I had an intense cold sweat, but figured that with my period and the fever, I was fighting something off. The next morning I remember dropping something on the floor. When I bent over to pick it up, my joints collapsed underneath my body weight. I could not get back up. It hurt. Then it hit me like a ton of bricks: Something was wrong, *really, really* wrong. Something foreign was in my body. I didn't know what it was, but it terrified me.

We arrived home late on the 23rd of June and called my pediatrician's office to make an appointment the next day. The fever hadn't subsided, the sweating had intensified, and my joint pain had become debilitating, to the point where walking was a huge task. I remember getting up from the chair in the waiting area and leaving a sweaty butt-cheek imprint. I giggle now thinking about it; it was not funny then. The doctor ordered some blood tests and said he would run them for rheumatoid arthritis, which matched my symptoms. (But even then, I knew my symptoms were also a match for leukemia, thanks to Googling before going to the doctor's office).

My labs were drawn, my results came back, and on June 25, 2013, the day after my mommy's birthday (bless her heart), I heard the words "You have cancer" for the first time. To make it extra special, I was told over the phone.

I do have to say, it was a relief to finally know what was wrong and that something was going to be done to make me feel better. My emotions were a mixture of confusion, relief, and *Wtf just happened?* I was admitted that very same day to the hospital to start chemo. My stay would last one week, during which I received my official diagnosis: very high-risk pre b-cell acute lymphoblastic leukemia.

In that first week, I would start chemo, my blood counts would bottom out, and I would have a PICC line placed into my left arm because my platelet count was not high enough for a port. I couldn't give you a whole lot of details beyond that because that first week was a blur.

During the induction phase of chemo (the first 28 days, essentially), the goal was to achieve remission. Following my inpatient stay, I continued to go to the outpatient clinic several times a week. Some days would be chemo days per protocol, others would be blood-count checks to determine whether I would need a transfusion of blood or platelets.

During my time at the pediatric outpatient clinic, there was something I found fascinating. If you observe the atmosphere there, you'll never know it's full of kids with very serious illnesses. These children are resilient. They might have pain or feel nauseated, but they're given some Zofran, some pain meds, and a small nap, and 30 minutes later, they're up and running and playing again (with their IV poles attached!). I couldn't feel sorry for myself, because I saw them. They fell, they got back up. I remember at one point accompanying an older family member to an outpatient cancer center for adults. I may or may not have gone on a tough day for the patients being treated, but I was slightly horrified at what I saw. Morale was low, there was not a whole lot of socializing, and people had a mopey, self-pitying attitude. You don't see a whole lot of that at the children's center, and that was very uplifting.

I achieved remission during induction. Per protocol, I still had to undergo the two-and-a-half-year treatment plan for my leukemia type. More than anything, to my understanding at least, this is done in order to prevent a relapse. The intensity of treatment depended on the phase that I was in. June to March of 2013, roughly the first eight months, were the most difficult, due to hair loss, weakness, and blood counts that left me immunocompromised. Once I began the maintenance phase, which was the longest (about 18 months), the infusions tapered to every two weeks, and then every month. My hair came back in, I gained *a lot* of weight, and I regained most of my strength. Although this was all great, something felt wrong. I felt like maybe it wasn't over and the worst was yet to come. I told my mom how I felt, and she told me that no matter what happened, I would never be alone because she was with me forever and always.

About one year into maintenance, I had a relapse scare, and we felt relief when that was ruled out. I knew my high-risk diagnosis meant a higher chance of relapse compared to someone with a low- or standard-risk diagnosis. Because of this, I asked my physician if I could keep my port in until I reached the 5-year post-diagnosis mark. I knew that it would require maintenance and monthly flushings, and I acknowledged that to her. She said no, the longer it was kept in, the higher the risk of infection.

I finally reached the end of my treatment and maintenance on November 4, 2015, two days before my 20th birthday. What better way to celebrate?

I continued to have follow-up appointments and lab draws biweekly, then monthly. My labs continued to improve. My doctor decided in January 2016 that it was time to have my port removed. I had labs drawn, had my pre-op appointment, and, on January 19, 2016, went forward with the removal.

About one week later, I started feeling unwell. I had flu-like symptoms, my head hurt, I had cold sweats, and my joints began to ache. I stayed in bed for several days and thought I was fighting something off. On February 3, I developed a fever, and none of my other symptoms subsided. I decided to give it a few days. My fever continued to increase and my joint pain was worsening, so I decided the next day to give my oncologist a call. She suggested I call my pediatrician and make a sick appointment. That didn't work, so I called my doctor back, and they gave me an appointment for February 5.

At the clinic, I was placed into an isolation bay in case I had the flu. I had my labs drawn, and it was maybe 10 minutes later that I saw my oncologist storm past my bay. Shortly after, she came back to my bay with my primary nurse, closed the door and curtain behind her, closed her eyes, and quietly whispered, "It's back."

There were a few seconds of silence, although it felt eternal. When my doctor opened her eyes, they were welled up. My mom's were too. I looked at both of them and told them that tears were the last thing I needed.

Remember how I had asked to keep my port in? Well, my doc looked me in the eye and said, "Did we really just take your port out?" *(Cue awkward silence.)*

Disclaimer: I absolutely love my oncologist. She is a sweetheart and one of my favorite people on this planet. That being said, I was not happy. I just shrugged my shoulders at her.

Just like with my first diagnosis, I was admitted that same day to begin treatment, this time for very high-risk refractory acute lymphoblastic leukemia. I had the option of taking the conventional treatment route but decided to participate in a clinical trial—because it might help me and also help someone else in the future. Even if it was not a success in my case, I'd have the gratification of knowing that I had done my part in allowing Western medicine to advance. I was OK with being a guinea pig. (The term "guinea pig" sounds kind of fucked-up, but that's how I felt in that moment, like I was helpless and had no other choice).

This protocol consisted of three phases. I would undergo the plan for the first phase, then await my biopsy results. Depending on those, I would either become ineligible or be randomized to two possible courses for the second part. It turned out I was randomized to the treatment course my doctor had hoped for: a continuous 28-day infusion of Blincyto (blinatumomab). I was the first patient at Children's Hospital of the King's Daughters (CHKD) to receive the drug.

Relapse treatment was rough. It was aggressive. My first treatment was a walk in the park compared to this. From February 5, 2016, to September 15, 2016, I spent 90% of my time in the hospital; not outpatient, but admitted and confined to the walls of a hospital bedroom. I was too sick to do anything, even if I had wanted to go home.

Besides having to deal with chemo and its side effects, somewhere along the way, because of my immunocompromised status, I would contract acute invasive fungal sinusitis. What is that, you ask? In a nutshell, my nose was quite literally black-molding from the inside out. In addition to my treatment protocol, I was having daily infusions of Amphotericin B, an antifungal dubbed *amphoterrible*—and I had to go to the OR several times a week for weeks. The OR visits were to have surgical debridements of my sinuses, to manually scrape and remove the mold. A combination of chemo, amphoterrible, and anesthesia fucked up my kidneys and temporarily set back my treatment. I was out of it a lot, but when I was awake, I tended to be and feel miserable. Shout out to my momma, my dad, my brother Victor, my amazing Tía Isabel and her wonderful kids, and Domingo, for making this a little bit less terrible. I love you guys more than you will ever know.

I was discharged from CHKD at the end of May, then went home for about 2 days before I had to head down to Duke for the next part of my treatment. Now that I had achieved remission, the plan was to prepare for a bone marrow transplant. Before we could begin the process to prepare, there was a laundry list of tests, tests, and more tests as part of the work up— to make sure, I guess you could say, that I was strong enough for a bone marrow transplant. I was in pretty bad shape. I went almost one whole month without any treatment while we decided what the next step was. Finally my doc at Duke sat down with me and said, "Look, your kidneys aren't in the best shape, but you're going on a month without chemo. A kidney we can replace. Another relapse will be harder to come back from." He then proceeded to tell me that he feared for my life if we didn't make a decision soon. It struck me right there: *I very well might not make it out alive.* It had never been said out loud, only implied. After that consult, I broke. I was scared. I wanted to scream. I didn't scream, though I did cry, like a baby. It was the only time I allowed myself to feel sorry for myself.

We decided, my doctor and I, that the best option was to begin the conditioning regimen for transplant. So I started conditioning. Eight TBI (total body irradiation) sessions, twice a day for four days. On the fourth day, I was admitted to the bone marrow unit after my morning session. Then followed four days of high-dose chemo, then one "rest" day, and on July 7, 2016, "day 0," I received my new cells. From there it was all a waiting game until I engrafted.

I was admitted July 1st and discharged September 15th, 2016, from the bone marrow unit at Duke. My discharge was the beginning of a long, isolated healing "journey" while my immune system recovered.

I try not to think about it a lot, but when I do think about everything my body was subjected to, I'm just like, *Holy shit, I'm a badass.* It took about a year after the transplant to start feeling significantly better and for me to regain some of my strength.

I now find myself in what you could call "survivorship" status, but it's anything but easy. Cancer left its mark, and I find myself wondering what to do with that. Medically I'm doing better, but the experience left my mind in a weird, fucked-up place. I just recently acknowledged that I need help and sought it out. I need to find myself before I can help anyone else.

When I was first diagnosed, I spoke with the priest from my parish and told him my faith was not in a good place. My family and friends kept their faith and prayed a whole lot for my healing, and I am thankful for that. But a lot of the things I saw messed me up. Sure I get to call myself a survivor, and everyone thanks God for that—but what about the others? The ones who didn't make it? Everyone talks about the miracle that I am because I beat the odds, so they thank God. Again, *what about the others?*

I saw a post some time ago on the Humans of New York Facebook page, and it really hit home with how I feel. It was from a pastor who said this: "I've been a deep believer my whole life…But it's just stopped making sense to me….It doesn't make sense to believe in a God that dabbles in people's lives. If a plane crashes and one person survives, everyone thanks God. They say, 'God had a purpose for that person. God saved her for a reason!' Do we not realize how cruel that is? Do we not realize how cruel it is to say that if God had a purpose for that person, he also had a purpose in killing everyone else on that plane? And a purpose in starving millions of children? A purpose in slavery and genocide? For every time you say that there's a purpose behind one person's success, you invalidate billions of people. You say there is a purpose to their suffering. And that's just cruel."

I could not have summarized my sentiments better. I just think it's fucked-up when someone says "God must have great plans for you," without thinking of what they are saying implies. Some say this thinking is flawed, but it's just how I feel. My priest did tell me that if I needed to vent, even if that meant using profanity at whatever I was mad at in a confidential way, he was more than happy to be that ear. I never did, though. What am I going to look like cussing out a priest, even if it's not directed at him?

Ultimately, I just feel guilty—guilty that I beat these incredible odds and others didn't, even those who had better odds than I did. I've not yet found a healthy way of coping with all of these feelings. During treatment, I remember breaking a whole lot of my mom's dinner plates (I blame it on the steroids though—damn 'roid rage). I shouldn't have done it, but I was angry. I still am sometimes. But it is what it is. I have to work on my relationship with the Big Guy. I feel like there is something missing in my life, and I think it's that. Faith has been a huge part of my upbringing, and it's just not there right now. I'm sure it'll come eventually. I do want to know what my "purpose" is, and I want to live a fulfilling life; but my body wasn't cured overnight, so my mind and soul won't be either.

When a Burden Becomes a Blessing

Name: Jayei H.

Location: Mississippi

Diagnosis: Anaplastic large-cell lymphoma; stage 4

Age at diagnosis: 29

Age now: 40

Before I was diagnosed with cancer, I feared death to the point where it was almost paralyzing to think about it. I had come to believe that I was going to be either blessed with great prosperity or experiencing tragedy in my life. I believed that because by age 29, nothing in life had been hard for me, ever. I never had to stress about family; I never had to stress about money. I did have health issues, like asthma and eczema, but that's nothing. You have an asthma attack, you go to the doctor. Your skin is messed up, you put cream on it. It wasn't anything that was stopping me from enjoying life. I was a military brat as a kid, so we traveled around a lot. School came easy; friendships came easy. I felt like this meant either I was destined for an easy life or I was being given this easy phase because I would have to buck up and get ready for a challenging future. So when I was diagnosed, it was eerie. I revisited all those thoughts. I figured that if tragedy was my fate, in the face of cancer, that equaled death. So I had this extreme anxiety about dying.

BEST ADVICE: During my last relapse, I told one of my nurses that I thought it might take me out. "So what?" she said. "What are you afraid of?" I told her I was afraid of dying. And she said, "Why?" At first I thought, *What's with this crazy lady? Somebody else can take my blood, 'cause I'm not feeling her.* But she went on to talk about her faith. She expressed such pleasure and joy in leaving this life so that she could meet her maker. The way she talked about it, her feelings were infectious. I left feeling, *Yeah, what am I worried about? I'm gonna be taken care of no matter what.*

At the time, I was finishing my sixth year as an elementary school teacher and counselor. I had my bachelor's degree in elementary education and my master's in counseling. I was still single, in very good health, pretty active. I traveled all the time—a trip every couple of months and an international trip once a year. I was quite happy.

When I got sick in the spring of 2008, it started like a cold, and I thought, *OK, I work in a school—the kids got me again.* But after a few weeks, I started to feel weak and thought it was developing into the flu or pneumonia.

My mom got worried, so she packed a bag and bought a one-way bus ticket to Atlanta. She had just retired the previous summer. She came with me to the doctor, and they said it was probably really bad pneumonia or the flu, or both. But while I was in the doctor's office, I had my first asthma attack in 20 years. My mom said, "I want her admitted to the hospital."

So they admitted me to ER. They ran scans and found fluid build-up around my heart. The ER doctor told me, "We need to do a quick surgery." I went from thinking I had a cold to having surgery, within like an hour. The surgery was to put a tube in to remove all that fluid. But what they still didn't know was that lymphoma was causing it, so from there things got progressively worse. Within a day or two, I was in intensive care, and I ended up staying there for three weeks. By that point, I was hooked up to so many machines, IVs, and needles. I had a breathing tube, a feeding tube, everything. It was in ICU that they finally saw the lymphoma on a scan. It was so aggressive that on the previous day's scan, they couldn't see it—but by the next day it was pervasive. My cancer was extremely aggressive, but, as my oncologist put it, also highly curable.

Before my family arrived, I had already started chemotherapy. I never got a chance to talk about fertility, because the situation was so dire that they had to move quickly. The change in my appearance and care was drastic. One day, the nurse I had seen when I first arrived came into my room. She greeted me cheerfully, then looked at my mom and said, "Oh, I know you. How is your daughter?" My mom looked at me and said, "Well, there she is." And the nurse replied, "Wait, you have two daughters here?" My mother told her, "No." The nurse looked at me and stopped talking. Finally she walked over and hugged me so tight. "Oh my gosh, we have been praying for you," she said. "I didn't recognize you, but I'm so happy to see you." It was an emotional moment.

The cancer had done a lot of damage to my heart before they found it. But when they started the chemo, I was very responsive to the treatment. It almost went away even with that first treatment, but I still finished the recommended regimen, which was continuous chemo at the hospital, 24 hours a day, for five days. Then I would go home for two weeks, then go back and do it all again. I did that six times. Needless to say, I did not go back to work, and I needed my mother to move in and take care of me. I did so well toward the end of my treatments that my doctor heeded my pleas and let me delay my last treatment by one week, to travel to Puerto Rico in celebration of my 30th birthday. I wrapped my hairless head in scarves, and of course we had a really good time.

Even though when chemo ended I was in complete remission, a team of oncologists recommended a stem cell transplant. I worked with a therapist to decide what to do, and I wrestled once again with fear of death. I also talked to my brother, who is devout in his faith. In the end, I came to terms with this notion—and it is just a notion—of dying. What happens when we die is ultimately beautiful, because no matter what you believe, if you're in pain, you're no longer going to be in pain. And if you are a believer, then you know you're going to a much better place. The people you leave behind, yes, they'll hurt—but they're also not going to worry about you anymore, and they'll be able to focus on themselves and heal. Cancer forced me to come to terms with death, but it was also part of maturing and growing in my faith. I don't have that paralyzing feeling anymore when I think about dying. I'm not afraid of it.

Ultimately I decided against the stem cell transplant. I felt like I had been through enough and that my faith was strong. I would be OK with my decision, even if the cancer recurred. But I didn't want to risk my life to cure something that there was a chance would never come back anyway.

Within a month or two of my last chemo treatment, I was back at work. I was doing well, and I continued to heal, thrive, and get stronger. I thought I'd had my brush with cancer and was done with it. But after four years in remission, I had a relapse. The cancer showed up under the skin in my right groin. So I went into chemotherapy again, successfully. But this time when they asked about a stem cell transplant, I said yes. Then I had to go into what I've heard called "salvage chemo," where they blast you with this ridiculously strong chemotherapy in preparation for the transplant. It's many times stronger than the average chemo, so it really wipes you and your entire immune system out. That's where the risk comes in. I think my chances were 60% for survival.

We decided to harvest my own stem cells rather than use a donor. I had so many that the nurses were taking bets on how many we would get. We got many more stem cells than I needed for the transplant! On my big day, a nurse inserted the stem cells, which is just like a transfusion. I had to spend the next three weeks in isolation, with daily full-day clinic visits to get fluids, see doctors, get blood work, answer a billion questions, and kick it with some awesome nurses and survivors. Again, although being in isolation wasn't fun, I responded really well to treatment. I went back into remission and stayed there for 11 months before I had another relapse. This time it was in my hip bone, and I was in extreme pain. I couldn't move up and down the stairs at my house. I needed someone caring for me all the time.

I agreed to do a second stem cell transplant, but this time an allogeneic transplant, which meant using donor cells. This is much more dangerous, and the risk is much higher for complications and death. I was willing, because I had done well with the first one, my insurance was on board, and I had a ready donor in my twin brother. (I'm a huge advocate for people to join the stem cell registry. You can save someone's life. I was blessed because I didn't have to wait to find a donor.)

So I signed up and again got my immune system blasted down to zero. My brother endured the process to harvest his stem cells for me. With any sibling, including a twin, unless you're an identical twin, there's only a one in four chance that they'll be a match for you. (Identical twins may not be the best donors for each other, because their cells might behave the same should there be a recurrence of disease.) It turned out that my twin was not only a match but a perfect 10/10 match.

The allogeneic stem cell transplant has more complications, so I was monitored more closely and had several hospitalizations. Any time my fever spiked, I had to be admitted. And just like with the earlier transplant, I limited my contact with people because I had no immune system to fight off disease. It's true isolation. I stayed in my house, I watched TV, I read, and I tried not to sulk.

What helped me most was when I started quilting by hand. I had read a book called *The Invention of Wings*, by Sue Monk Kidd, who also wrote *The Secret Life of Bees*. *The Invention of Wings* was about an African American woman who got by during slavery because she was an extremely talented seamstress. The book gives these amazing descriptions of her phenomenal quilts. I like crafts, and I'd liked to sew as a kid. So I asked my mom if she would teach me how to quilt. She went and bought a whole bunch of materials for me, since I couldn't go out to shop for them myself. She picked out fabric in beautiful, bright colors that totally speak to her personality, and I liked them a lot. She laid the materials out in front of me, showed me with one or two stitches what to do, and let me take it from there. At the end, she helped me bind the quilt, and we finished it on the machine.

Quilting by hand got me through that time. I had a sewing machine, but that wasn't what I needed. I needed to be consumed by a task, using my hands to move that needle through the material, with my headphones on, listening to some music, with light from a table lamp. This was therapeutic for me. It saved my sanity. Sometimes neuropathy got in the way, but if it hurt too much I would just put the sewing down and come back to it later. I never quilted for more than an hour at a time. It was fascinating to watch one 4x4 inch square grow into a twin-size comforter at my own hands! The brightness of the colors my mom picked lifted my spirits while I was on isolation. Hours and hours of sewing produced a beautiful quilt that I find so much comfort in, even to this day, years later. My recovery was eased with this project of mine, and I am grateful for it. I wished I had endeavored such a task during my first transplant. I still machine quilt a little bit, but not as much.

I was so sure after my second stem cell transplant that I was done with cancer forever. But just a month later, in August of 2014, I developed a knot on the inner thigh of my right leg. The knot was so hard that when they tried to biopsy it, the first nurse couldn't even get the needle through, and the second one had to push with all her might. I was numbed, so I just felt a lot of tugging and pressure. But watching them, I was thinking, *This can't be good.*

I remember the moment they came to get me to tell me the news. The doctor found me in the chemo room and asked to talk to me. I followed him back to the consultation room. I have a love/hate relationship with those rooms. I've gotten some great news in them, and I've gotten some horrible news in them. Walking, pushing my IV pole, I looked back at my mom, and we locked eyes. Then I just shook my head back and forth. I knew it was bad. She started following me, and in her eyes, I could see she had no idea what to say or do.

In the room, we sat down, and the doctor said it was lymphoma again. I looked at him and said, "Is this the beginning of the end?"

He looked back and said, "I don't know."

I started crying, and I lay my head on my mom's lap. One by one, all the nurses came in to love on me, hug on me, pray with me, and encourage me. Still, that moment was the first time when I felt completely helpless and almost hopeless.

The doctor said, "We're not giving up. We have a few options, and I want to talk to you about them. Number one, that cancer is at the surface of your skin, so we can put you back on chemo and closely monitor it. We can see what it's doing." This is the first time that my doctors could visibly see the lymphoma presenting; before, it had been subcutaneous. Every day they photographed and measured it. My doctor recommended I take what they call a booster—another dose of my brother's stem cells—which they had on ice. So we did that. I say we because we are a team. I always say, "We beat cancer," because I have the best support system.

The doctors put me back on immunosuppression so that my brother's cells could do the work and my own cells would be less likely to attack my new cells. Immunosuppression helped my body not to reject his cells. I did well after the booster. In December of 2014 I had my last round of chemotherapy, and by January I had another clean bill of health. I haven't had another relapse since. I'm more than four years cancer free, in a battle that has been 11 years altogether.

Last August, three big things happened: I finished my PhD in Educational Theory and Practice from the University of Georgia; I was released from my oncologists' care; and I turned 39 years old. It took me 10 years to finish my doctorate, because of all my relapses and subsequent leaves of absence from the university. I had to jumpstart my postgraduate studies a couple of times, but I walked for graduation in December. I'm now in a new job, working for the first time in four years. It's at a summer camp for gifted high schoolers. Soon I'll start a job as a learning coordinator at a local elementary school.

Over the years, medical bills took the money I used to spend on vacations and drained my savings. But that didn't stop me from traveling. I was obsessed with finding resources to help offset my costs, and I ended up finding out about many opportunities to travel and becoming part of the awesome young-adult survivor community I'd had no idea even existed. Over the years since, I've had the opportunity to participate and volunteer for several programs that believe in building an active life after cancer. It has been so rewarding to receive this type of support and be able to give back. I have also met many amazing young, strong people determined to not let cancer define them or their lives. They have taught me so much about life, and I now live to the fullest each day, with greater intention.

Since I started working, I have been able to climb out of some of the debt created by medical bills and educational expenses. This chapter of my life feels like I am in more control, but I want to learn to fully relinquish control to a higher power. Slowly, I am learning to keep God first, and that helps me not to worry so much. I want to be a contributing member of this exclusive club of survivorship, instead of running from it. Opportunities to share my story feel less like a burden than they used to. And what a beautiful feeling— when a burden becomes a blessing.

Silver Comet & the Tour de Pink

Name: Tamika Partridge

Town: Newnan, Georgia

Diagnosis: Breast cancer; ER-, PR-, HER2- ("triple negative")

Age at diagnosis: 37

Age now: 42

I am a single working mom. When I was diagnosed, my son was about 4 and in his first year of kindergarten. My daughter was in her first year of college. My first priority after my diagnosis was to make sure my kids kept the same lifestyle they'd had. I wanted to coordinate everything myself. In my family, I'm the person everybody goes to when they need everything, so I didn't have anybody to help me.

My mom is a two-time breast cancer survivor, and I knew I carried the BRCA2 mutation. When I was diagnosed, I had been in surveillance for two years, alternating a mammogram and breast MRI every six months. Every time I went, my anxiety kicked up—so much so that I had missed my last visit. I didn't want to have the BRCA testing to start with. I put it off for so long after my mom and my sister did it. Like I said, my mom's a two-time cancer survivor. She had genetic testing after her second diagnosis, and my sister had it at the same time. I knew both of them had the mutation. But I always said I didn't want anybody to tell me anything that I could die from.

I got the news of my diagnosis in a phone call. But there had been something about the biopsy—I knew bad news was coming. It was the worst biopsy I had ever had in my life. It hurt so bad I cried on the table. I just knew it was cancer. I was just waiting for the call to confirm it. Still, you're never prepared.

BEST ADVICE: Survivors told me, don't take your nausea medicine when you get nauseous—that's too late. Take it before. The bottle doesn't say that. It says "Take as needed" or "One every four hours." I would start my nausea medication maybe three days prior to my chemo and then take it around the clock. That way, it was always in my system, and if I did get a little nauseous, it wasn't bad. I never threw up the entire time I was on chemo.

I work in health care, doing insurance and billing in OB/GYN. So I knew which were the good breast cancer surgeons, from doing referrals. I didn't know anything about oncologists. My main concern was making sure I got the best care. I was fortunate in that my home is five miles from the

Cancer Treatment Center of Atlanta, which is actually 20 miles south of Atlanta in Newnan. I ended up doing chemo first. I had Adriamycin and Cytoxan, followed by Carboplatin and Taxol. My surgery choice was pretty easy—being BRCA2 positive, I chose mastectomies. Being BRCA2 also means you're at a higher risk for cervical cancer, so I decided to have a hysterectomy at the same time. I didn't want to go through multiple surgeries. Surgery lasted about eight hours, and they put the expanders in too. It was hard because my mom wasn't there with me. She was in the hospital herself at the same time, for surgery. She ended up in the ICU but then was moved to a rehabilitation center. She somehow managed to get out in time to come see me right after I came out of surgery.

After I had expanders placed, it was like my body rejected them. My incisions kept opening. I would be at three weeks, looking like I was completely healed, and then by the beginning of the fourth week, they were opening up and I was going back to surgery. I probably did about five surgeries after the mastectomy. Finally, they had to remove the expanders so I could start radiation. I did it every day for five weeks. I had to remain flat for at least six months, I think it was. I went to Hawaii that way. Finally, in April of 2016, I chose to have a DIEP-flap surgery, which is what I'd wanted to do all along. This surgery ended up being 15 hours, and the recovery was worse than for the mastectomy and hysterectomy. I was driving in two weeks after those. But DIEP-flap surgery really put me down. I hardly moved for four to five weeks. I remember being in ICU right after, for about four days. I remember singing that song—you know that song that says, "You all going make me lose my mind up in here"? My son was one of the biggest supporters during my recovery. I really didn't have to explain a whole lot. He was just like my baby.

Since then, I've been under surveillance because of my triple-negative pathology. The first five years, you're under close surveillance. Actually, the first year, you're under *really* close surveillance. I think you go every three months. After that, you graduate to every six months.

To be honest, throughout my treatments, I've been very happy. My treatment was a lot different from a lot of people's because I stayed active. I worked. I stayed busy.

I got involved with the Young Survival Coalition thanks to one of my friends who was running the Face 2 Face support group for YSC locally. She asked me to come and be a part of it with her. I ended up becoming a Face 2 Face leader for South Atlanta.

Then YSC had a conference in Atlanta, and I went. The sisterhood with YSC is great. When you go to a conference, it changes your life. YSC is a stepping stone as far as meeting people. You can go out to a YSC conference by yourself and, I guarantee, you're going to come out with 10 friends or more.

At the YSC conference, I learned about the annual Tour de Pink fundraising bike ride. It's a 200-mile ride, spread over three days. I also learned that there's a company, Live, that works with YSC to give bikes to survivors. Being me, I applied for a bike! I never thought I would get one. But one day, I had my phone in my hand, and I saw an email notification come across the top that said, "Congratulations." I'm like, "For what?" I opened the email and was like, "Oh, my God. You've got to be kidding." I got the bike. Part of keeping the bike is that you have to commit to riding in the Tour de Pink and raising $2,500 to do the ride.

I figured, hey, I need a new lifestyle. I used to be a runner prior to diagnosis, but at this point I wasn't doing anything. Maybe this could be my new norm. I got into it. I didn't train very well for my first ride, but I trained with this guy, Scott, who had ridden many of the Tour de Pinks. I would meet him and ride on Silver Comet, my bike. He would tell me, "You got this."

I think my longest consecutive ride was 30 miles or 40 miles during my first Tour de Pink. Scott said, "You can do it. It's a piece of cake." When I got to the finish line, it was the best thing ever. After that first ride, I made a commitment that my way of giving back to breast cancer would be to ride every year. Between the two years I've ridden so far, I've raised around $6,000.

Then I became a state leader for YSC. I meet with health-care providers and update them with new information about YSC and about breast cancer. A lot of people reach out to state leaders, asking us to share our stories. At health fairs, we have a table dedicated to YSC. I love it.

The reason I learned about YSC was that when I met with my first breast surgeon, before I got accepted into the treatment center, a nurse-navigator walked into the room holding a binder. She gave it to me and was like, "There are people just like you." It was all young people with breast cancer. I said, "I've never heard of this."

I've also been a part of a patient-advisory board for triple-negative people for AstraZeneca, the pharmaceutical company. They're working on an immunotherapy clinical trial for triple-negative patients. And I work with ABCD: After Breast Cancer Diagnosis. I'm a mentor with them. I'm also a "Cancer Fighter" with Cancer Treatment Centers of America.

I'll continue to ride in the Tour de Pink. I'll continue to advocate. With ABCD, I'm mentoring four people right now, and I will continue to mentor and connect with a lot of different people outside of that. One of my ABCD mentees was matched with me because she wanted to talk to another single mom who went through breast cancer, to talk about how to take care of her kids while she's in treatment.

I got through it with help from my family—including relatives who have died. My grandmother and my aunt were two of the strongest people I knew. My aunt died of liver cancer not too long before my diagnosis. My grandmother died a couple of years previous to that. I was very close to them. Just being around them all my life—they always taught me to keep pushing and not to give up. When I went through it, I always carried their strength with me.

The only thing cancer made me do differently is, I live more intentionally now. I don't put things off. If I get a chance to travel, I travel. I make sure I'm enjoying my life.

I am starting a nonprofit, Mom Survived More. It's based on my experience as a single parent who went through breast cancer. In order to keep up with things during treatment and without changing our lifestyle, I had to burn through all our savings. Now we have debt and have had to downgrade by moving to an apartment, among other things.

Not everybody has savings, and my goal is to be able to provide some financial support to single parents. My son, for example, plays a lot of sports. Some parents may need help paying for sports registration. My son went to private school and needed a school uniform. Christmastime came around—parents may need something for Christmas. And then I thought of other things based on where my daughter was at the time, entering her first year of college. We want to provide care baskets and other little things that new college kids need.

Right now we're starting however we can, in small ways. It takes time to build a nonprofit, but the name's out there. I have a Facebook page, so go like it! It's Mom Survived More.

Sticking It to Throat Cancer

Name: Hannah Wright

Town: Shelbyville, Kentucky

Diagnosis: Throat cancer, stage 4

Age Diagnosed: 26

Age Now: 28

Before I got cancer, I was living at home with my mom, if that tells you anything. I was struggling to find who I was as a person and what I wanted to be doing with my life.

Soon after I was diagnosed, I started a journal. I wrote in it every day of my treatment. The first day read: *July 11th was the day that I found out that I have throat cancer. The day that will forever change my life. I am about to embark on the hardest journey, but I have to stay strong—not only for myself but for my loved ones. This is an obstacle that life has thrown at me. I will prevail and conquer this. I just have to keep saying that, over and over in my head. I can't help but think: Why me? Is God trying to teach me a lesson, or is it to prove to myself that I am strong? I've always had self-doubt. This is a moment to prove to myself that I can overcome the hardest tasks—but like they say, cancer has no prejudice.*

BEST ADVICE: Look on the brighter side of things.

I had started smoking cigarettes when my grandpa, who was like a dad to me, was sick with cancer. It was stress relief. I wish I'd never done that—but cigarettes aren't how I got throat cancer, although they probably delayed my diagnosis. I got cancer from HPV. Usually HPV causes cervical or ovarian cancer, but in 15% of cases, it causes throat cancer.

I had the Gardasil vaccine as a teenager, but it's likely I got HPV before that. I've been in therapy, so I'm open now about the trauma I experienced as a child. When I was 7, my dad raped me. The abuse lasted until I was 11. I've had issues with men my whole life. The only men I was OK around were my grandfather and my brother. Other than that, I was not having it being around men—until I met my fiancé in 2009 at a friend's party. We were drawn to each other right away.

My first symptom of cancer was that when I swallowed, it felt like I was swallowing a rock. For months, my primary-care doctor was convinced I had bronchitis. But then one night I woke up gasping for air. I was turning blue. My mom rushed me to the ER, and they had to do an emergency tracheostomy. I woke up and found out I had cancer. The tumor had squeezed my vocal chords closed. It was the size of a strawberry, which is really big considering the area. They said that I had had cancer for about a year prior to being diagnosed, and it had spread to one of my lymph nodes in my left jaw.

They told my mom before I even woke up from the surgery, so she was already freaking out. She's my Number One—my biggest supporter in my life. She's always been a single parent, and my being sick was super hard on her. That week I was in the hospital, my dad had the audacity to try to come see me. My mom kicked him out with curses and threats. She was like, "If you come in this hospital, you will be in a room." She went straight *mom*, and I was so proud of her.

My doctor said, "All right, so here are your two options. We can either take out your vocal box completely—which we would have already done if you were in yours 40s or 50s, without giving you an option—or we can do chemo and radiation." Obviously, I took the second option. I did six weeks of radiation on my neck, and then I did four or five different chemo injections. I had this little purple thing they put over your trach to help you talk. It helps you learn how to breathe again and how to swallow. If I took it off, I couldn't have a drink, because I could get fluid in my lungs.

My treatment was in the middle of summer, so it was hot as heck. I couldn't go outside because I couldn't breathe with the humidity. I basically had to stay in my bedroom with an AC unit on full blast. I was always freezing, so I developed a sock obsession, and people got me like 70 pairs. I was glued to my Fire Stick watching *Game of Thrones*. I would go outside at night when it was cooler, just to get out of the house for a minute.

The first few weeks of radiation were all right. It didn't really hurt my neck much. I was able to eat. But toward the end, my neck was black from my ears to my collarbone. I ate through a feeding tube for the last three weeks. Then I ended up getting a staph infection and MRSA in my feeding-tube area. Fortunately I have state Medicaid, which covered all my medical bills, including all the medicine.

There was a humidifier I had to wear on my neck, over my trach, to keep it from getting dry. If the mucus inside the trach gets dry, it cuts off your airway. It got to the point where if it was dry, I would have to stick this long rubber thing down my neck and suction it out. That was the worst part. It made me gag. That was a nasty part of cancer, you know. Everybody has nasty parts. You never realize how much drainage you get from your nasal cavity and your neck. I was like, "Whoa." It's a lot.

My grandma drove me 40 minutes each way to my appointments every day. She's a hard nut to crack. My grandfather passed away from brain cancer in 2013. He was my surrogate dad and her best friend, her everything. Grandma didn't take my being sick too well because she went through it with him. When I got sick, she was helping to take care of me plus taking care of my twin cousins. My siblings would watch the kids while she helped me. So it was a team effort, really.

If it weren't for my family, I probably wouldn't have done as well as I did. They pick my spirits up. Our family wasn't as connected as it should have been, but when I got sick, it brought everybody together. My grandpa wasn't there, but I feel like he was fighting along with me. I have a picture of him over my bed. I just feel like he was helping me through it. My cousin works at a doctor's office and deals with people with a variety of serious illnesses. She said, "Just keep a smile on your face, and when the dark seems to surround you, keep calm and stay strong—you will carry on." That always stuck with me.

My younger sister, who is 22, started a GoFundMe for me. We raised $2500. It helped a lot. She's my best friend, there for me every step of the way. She would take me out every now and then for a drive. We did art projects together to pass the time—drawing, bracelets, coloring books. I have too many coloring books! We made friendship bracelets with whatever colors a family member wanted. The little kids loved them and would help make them, too. We made pictures and other things to decorate my bedroom. We were trying to make it bright and colorful because I had so much medical equipment in there.

The whole time I was like, *Just keep swimming*—like Dory the fish. *I can do this*. But it would get really dreary at times. I tried not to let it get me down, but sometimes it would. I already had PTSD because of what I went through as a child, and during my illness it turned into bipolar disorder. Medicaid allowed me to see mental-health practitioners and get on medicine. During the worst time, I was wanting to overdose and hurt myself. If my mom hadn't been there for me, I probably would have done it, honestly. I had liquid Percocet and was injecting it into my feeding tube, trying to numb myself to everything that was happening. But I realized what I was doing and turned to my mom. I told her to take the medicine away and give me one dose at a time.

My fiancé also took care of me—everyone did. He found mobile humidifiers on Amazon, so we could go places without my trach drying out. He took me to the state fair, and with that thing I could walk around and do everything I wanted to. It all started to get easier once we figured out different ways to get around complications.

I'm someone who is really spunky and quirky and "out there." I was the same way when I was sick. I had my hard days and my happy-go-lucky days. Seeing me with my humidifier and my trach, everybody in the community was like, "What the heck's going on?" Especially kids, because they don't understand—but even adults. I'd see people staring at me, but I wasn't going to let it get me down. I already had too much stuff getting me down from my past.

Since diagnosis, I have completely changed my demeanor. I used to be a pushover. Now, I'm sticking it to people. I'm not letting anybody walk all over me and treat me like crap anymore. Cancer kind of made me turn over a new leaf. I took on that challenge that I wrote in my journal on day 1—to prove to myself I could overcome any situation.

My trach got taken out in November, two days before Thanksgiving. I've had it out for five months. The radiation shrank everything really fast. It got the tumor and got the cancer out of my lymph nodes. I was really surprised. I was diagnosed July 11, 2017, and I found out I was in remission on December 20th. That was my Christmas gift.

When my treatment was over, I was depressed and scared. I was like, "How's it gonna be from here on out?" Before cancer, I hadn't been on a good path. I didn't know which way was up. I was bouncing from job to job and emotionally unstable. But cancer opened my eyes. I had to grow up and get my ass in gear. If I was going to get a second chance, I needed to do it right.

Despite the fear, good things were happening. After my last radiation appointment, at the hospital, my fiancé asked me to marry him. He was there with a bouquet of flowers. It was so sweet. It helped me so much to know that somebody would still love me, even the way I look, even through everything I went through.

I'm going to be a stepparent. He just started kindergarten. I'm focusing on that—making a family and taking care of myself. I've been working out like crazy. A few weeks ago I went back to work. I feel like a new person. I still need to have my fertility checked, because they said there's the chance I might have issues. I hope I can have biological kids. I would love to have one. But, you know, stuff happens.

Before I got sick, I was terrified of everything. After all this, I feel like I'm fearless. This is the happiest I've been in my life. Yes, it happened. I got sick. It was terrible. But it changed me for the good.

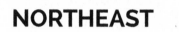

NORTHEAST

I Am Not Angelina:
One Woman's Choice to Keep Her Breasts
. . . .

Name: Jordana Bales

Town: New York, NY

Diagnosis: Breast cancer; stage 0 (DCIS) and stage 1; BRCA2 positive

Age When Diagnosed: 42

Age: 48

Jordana's contribution is an essay she wrote about her decision not to have a mastectomy.

I'd always feared cancer. It ran on both sides of my family. As a 4th- grader, when my friends worried about boys and clothes, I would lay awake at night worrying about cancer. My father has several first cousins with a breast cancer gene mutation who suggested I should be tested. In 2007, when I found out I had the mutation (BRCA2), I felt relief. Now cancer couldn't surprise me!

What did surprise me was the pressure I felt to cut off my breasts. "You're a smart girl—I know you'll make the right decision," said Dr. M., my early-surveillance doctor. The "right decision" according to him was a double mastectomy, for a small (less than 1 cm) group of stage 0 (DCIS) cancer cells.

Some people consider DCIS "precancerous." In Europe, they don't treat it. They adopt a "wait and see" approach. Because I am an educated woman who respected her doctor's opinion, I spent about two months trying to convince myself that a double mastectomy was the answer. I would finally come to realize that keeping my breasts was actually the right decision for me.

During my years of screening (alternating mammograms and MRIs every 6 months, plus manual breast exams every 6 months—my breasts were getting more attention than Kim Kardashian's!), I expected that I would develop cancer. After all, the documentation I received with my genetic-testing results stated that "80% of BRCA-positive women will get breast cancer by age 70"—a prediction that has since been significantly decreased. As a daughter of a statistician, I understood the odds.

Yet I never wanted to remove my breasts prophylactically. When Dr. M. mentioned it to me originally (prior to my cancer diagnosis), I quickly dismissed the suggestion. It seemed barbaric and dramatic. Now, with a diagnosis of stage 0 (DCIS) cancer, I was planning to do it. But it didn't feel right.

Thus began a mission to convince myself that a double mastectomy was, as my 68-year-old male primary-care physician put it, a "no brainer." I spoke to many women who had undergone the surgery. They talked about the relief they experienced (I wanted relief!). They spoke about making the "right" decision in order to be around for their children (I had two young daughters—I should be responsible!). I went to a breast cancer support group where the leader, a kind and knowledgeable woman, repeatedly said, "We all can make choices in our treatment—except you, Jordana" (my only choice, she believed, was to remove my breasts and the future possibility of another cancer). I joined a group of "previvors"—women with the gene mutation who had not gotten cancer. Their topic of conversation was the type of surgery they were planning to prevent cancer (I wanted to prevent cancer!).

I had phone conversations with friends and family in which I attempted to convince them—really trying to convince myself—that this was necessary. I would say, "If I don't do it and down the road I am dying from breast cancer, I'll wish I'd done everything I could have. This is the time to do everything." Or I would point out, "My daughters will never see their mother get breast cancer."

But it wasn't down the road—it was now. And I already had breast cancer. And I wasn't really scared of dying from it. I never saw any women in my family suffer with breast cancer. I did not witness my grandma, mother, aunt, or sister lose their hair, their breasts, their life. I got the mutation from my Dad, who got it from his Dad. My father's sister, my aunt, did not have it. I have no sisters. None of the BRCA-positive women in my family who have had cancer died from it. And most of them did not have double mastectomies.

It was time to find out the facts. I wanted to know the actual chances of reoccurrence and of death. My surgeon told me that removing my breasts decreased the risk of a future breast cancer but did not significantly reduce the risk of death from the diagnosis I had. I went to a genetic counselor and was told I had only a 15% chance of developing breast cancer again in the next 10 years.

Why was I removing my breasts if there was an 85% chance that I would not get breast cancer in the next ten years? And even if I did get it, my chance of dying from it was only 10-20%. My only purpose in removing my breasts was to avoid dying of breast cancer in the future—but there was only a 3% chance that would happen. I decided I could live with that.

I chose to be aggressive with the cancer I did have, rather than the cancer I did not have. Further tests showed that in addition to the stage 0 cells, I also had some stage 1 triple-negative cells. To treat them, I had both chemotherapy and radiation. I spent 2013 dealing with this cancer. When my friends wanted to celebrate the end of my treatment, I was hesitant. I continue to get screened and think there is a fair possibility cancer will be discovered again. But that thought scares me far less than the thought of removing my breasts.

Should cancer be in my future, I will deal with it. I can always rethink my choice. But for now, my breasts and I are content with this decision.

I am not Angelina Jolie. I am not Christina Applegate. I am not a hero. I am a member of another group of strong women whose stories aren't being told: Women who also looked at facts and statistics and decided that keeping their breasts was their right decision. Women should not be made to feel that one option is "smarter" or more "heroic" than another. Neither choice is a "no brainer."

Blindsided & Buttered Toast

· ·

Name: Eden Bertrang

Town: Brooklyn, New York

Diagnosis: Sinonasal undifferentiated carcinoma (SNUC) with neuroendo-crine features; stage 4

Age at diagnosis: 29

Age now: 40

In 2006, I was living in New York City and starting a new career as a birth doula—a trained and experienced birth coach. By 2007, I had saved up enough money from waitressing to start my own business and was attending three to four births per month. I was also teaching yoga—prenatal and post-natal yoga, mostly. By 2008, my husband Jyota and I had been married for about two years, and I was living what would be considered a very healthy lifestyle. I was not a smoker, I drank only the occasional glass of wine, and I was mostly a vegetarian. I didn't have any obvious risk factors for head-and-neck cancer.

About a year before I was diagnosed, I was babysitting for a friend of mine and slipped on a toy car. I went up into the air, landed on the kid's drum set, and ended up lacerating my lip and breaking my nose. I had to go to the hospital, where a plastic surgeon gave me stitches and told me my nose would heal on its own.

BEST ADVICE: Surround yourself with advocates. Take friends and family members to appointments, so that they can provide a second set of ears during conversations with your care team. My stepmother brought a book to all appointments and took notes. She then had the great idea of leaving the book with me, so that my friends could write down what was said during medical consults. That way, we were all literally on the same page!

It didn't—at least, not completely. All through the summer and fall, I had bleeding on and off. I finally called the surgeon and said, "The bleeding isn't quite resolved, and it's always in the left nostril." He said, "Well, healing can be slow. That's to be expected. Don't worry about it." Then in the winter, I was feeling a lot of pressure behind my eyes and, again, having in-termittent nosebleeds. I went to an ophthalmologist who checked for pressure and said, "No, there's no pressure behind your eyes. Don't worry about it— you have perfect eyesight!"

A couple more months went by, and I started having swelling around my eyes and sinus congestion. I went to a clinic and said, "I'm feeling kind of stuffed up, and I'm losing my sense of smell." The doctor said, "Oh, you probably have a sinus infection. We'll give you some antibiotics." But antibiotics didn't make it better. Then it was the spring, and the doctor said, "This underlying inflammation you've had in your sinuses has probably led to severe allergic rhinitis"—so he prescribed a nasal spray with antihistamines. When I started having really big nosebleeds, the doctor said, "That's a side effect of the nasal spray. Speak to the nurse about how to apply it." I followed her instructions, but the bleeding continued.

By the summer of 2008, I couldn't breathe out of my nose at all. It was chronically plugged up, and I was beginning to feel more tired. Then I went to Tennessee, to the Farm—a commune that is famous now for the resurgence of midwifery in the United States. I went there to study with Ina May Gaskin, a renowned midwife and author—and while I was there, my eyes started to swell, to the point that I looked like I had black eyes. One of the midwives said, "You know, some people get those when they have really bad allergies. They're called 'allergy shiners.'" The antihistamines and nasal sprays clearly weren't helping, and neither were the homeopathic and herbal remedies I had started to take.

When I got back to New York, it had been 20 days since I had seen my husband. When Jyota saw me, he said, "Honey, you don't even look like you." I said, "What do you mean?" He answered, "Your eyes look like they're spread apart. You look really, really sick." I went back to the doctor and he said, "You should get a CT scan. Since you don't have insurance, you're going to have to wait for an appointment through the subsidized program at the hospital." My appointment was set for October 31st. This was in August.

A couple of weeks later, I had a seizure. I came home from attending a birth, took a shower, lay down—and then I wet the bed! I got up, feeling disoriented. I remember getting to my phone and not knowing how it worked. I saw a green button and thought, *Green means "go."* I pushed it and the phone called my husband, because he was the last person I had called.

"I think I just had a seizure," I told him. Of course he came home, and we went to a neighborhood doctor who said, "I don't think you had a seizure. There's nothing about you that makes me think you've had a seizure." After that I went to my acupuncturist, and we did a treatment. Then I vomited bile all night long.

On a friend's recommendation, I went to New York Eye and Ear Hospital in Manhattan the next morning. I was bleeding from my nose and occasionally vomiting. I had patches of numbness in my face. An ENT in the walk-in clinic looked up my nose with a scope and said, "You have these little Schneiderian polyps. I'll need to do a biopsy. They are only malignant about 10% of the time—and you're young and healthy. There's no reason to think that you would have cancer. We'll also have to do a CT scan. We'll find out how far back they go, and then we can remove them for you."

I went for the scan, and the technician said, "We'll call you back in 24 to 48 hours." Instead, the hospital called me back four hours later and said, "You have to come back." I responded, "Well, today is not really a good day for me because I'm working."

Then I thought to myself, *If they're calling back an uninsured woman and telling her to come back to the hospital to meet with three doctors, it's bad, right? It has to be bad.* That, by the way, was the other stressful thread through all this: I didn't have health insurance. My husband and I were both freelancers, and we just couldn't afford it.

I said to Jyota, "I think I have cancer." I was right.

The kind of cancer I turned out to have—sinonasal undifferentiated carcinoma—is a rare and aggressive form of cancer in the lining of the nose or sinuses. People who are diagnosed with nasal and sinus cancers are typically men in their 60s who smoke and/or drink heavily. Woodworkers and nickel-factory workers can also be at a higher risk. That's why it was missed. Even though I was showing many textbook signs of sinus cancer, no one was looking for SNUC in a healthy 29-year-old. No one gives a 29-year-old doula/yoga instructor a CT scan when she has signs of a sinus infection or allergies. By the time I was diagnosed, the cancer had spread through all of my sinuses. It was stage 4.

My reaction to the diagnosis surprised the doctors. I told them upfront that I wasn't sure I wanted to be treated at all. My mother was diagnosed with breast cancer when I was 9 and had a mastectomy around my 10th birthday. She then underwent chemotherapy and radiation—this was in 1989. The cancer went into remission, and she had a prophylactic mastectomy to make sure that she wouldn't have cancer again. But three years later, the cancer metastasized. She had a recurrence in her lungs just before I turned 13. When I was 15, she died; and even though I was devastated, I was relieved. Her treatments had gone on for far too long, and it had been traumatic to watch her suffer.

By the time of my diagnosis, I couldn't breathe through my nose, I was having consistent bleeding, I had no sense of smell, and one eye—my right eye—had been lifted out of its socket, altering my vision. Because I had so much pressure on my frontal lobe, I was having impulse-control issues, and my executive function was compromised. I knew that I wasn't afraid of death. I was definitely afraid of suffering, though—not just for myself, but for the effect my suffering would have on my family. I didn't want that for my family and friends, or for myself. I was pretty clear about that—I didn't want to prolong my life through treatment if it meant having a really poor quality of life. The doctors didn't think I knew what I was saying.

One of the oncologists said, "Nine out of 10 people will respond to therapy." I knew "respond" didn't mean they were cured, but she also said that although it was an intense treatment, she had patients who got through it. She explained, "We have some people who've been living for a while with the disease. They still have cancer, but they're living comfortably with cancer. The drugs that we have now are not like the drugs your mother took."

The other oncologist said, "I respect your choice not to accept treatment, but you don't have that much time to decide. If you don't choose treatment, you'll be in palliative care within a couple of weeks."

Ultimately, I decided to accept treatment. I think it was partly because I knew that my father, who flew in from Canada to be with me during my first round of chemo, didn't want to lose me. And I knew that my husband wanted me to at least give treatment a try. We agreed that I would stop if I was suffering. And then, there was a moment for me—a shift that took place—when I decided that if I was going to do the treatment, I was going to get through it and survive.

My first chemo treatment was almost my last. My kidneys lost their ability to regulate my salt, and I had an episode of severe hyponatremia and was transferred to the ICU. My stepmother flew in and began to play an important role in advocating for me. I ended up staying in the hospital for 10 days.

I was home for only four days before starting the protocol again. Because the initial diagnosis was stage 4, the doctors told me I would have to do three rounds of chemotherapy, each four days long and 10 days apart, which they hoped would shrink the tumor by 50%. I'd follow up with 15 high-dose radiation treatments, which would take care of another 25% of it. Finally I would have surgery, with a skull-based surgeon, an ENT, and a neurologist present.

What ended up happening, though, was that the chemotherapy actually knocked out almost all of the cancer. Even without scans, I knew I was getting better with the chemo. I knew it because I could hear it in my voice. Since I couldn't go anywhere during chemo, I had decided to take voice lessons again. It had been a couple of years since I had actively pursued music—I'd actually moved to New York to go to theater school, and music had been a major part of my life, both professionally and recreationally, for many years. When my focus shifted to doula work, my involvement in music fell by the wayside; but during chemo, I went to lessons twice a week. As time went on, my voice became less nasal and more resonant, because the tumors were shrinking and I had more space in my sinuses. I was finally starting to breathe through my nose again. I had lost all my hair, my eyebrows, my eyelashes— but my voice was coming back, and I knew I was getting better.

When it was time for radiation, I asked about side effects from treatment. The doctor said, "Well, you can have some burning on your skin, and it can really make you feel fatigued." I said I wanted to know about the long-term side effects. My doctor was like, "You really just need to focus on living." And I said, "I understand that, but what are the long-term side effects?"

He said, "You'll have ongoing dry mouth. It's unclear whether you'll regain your sense of smell...probably not."

And I was like, "What else?"

He said, "Well, your pituitary gland will probably be shot. And...we're gonna have to watch your eyes closely." I asked if I was going to need glasses.

"No, I mean we have to make sure that you keep your vision," he said.

Thinking of the eye that had been pushed out of its socket, I said, "Oh, you mean I might lose vision in my right eye?"

"No," he said. "You could go blind in both eyes."

And I was like, *What?* I couldn't believe this had not been made more clear to me! Finally, he explained that it was impossible to shield the optic nerves from radiation. At that point I said, "I'm not really sure I understand the benefits. I mean, I feel great after the chemotherapy. The cancer has resolved. Why would I follow up with radiation if it's gonna make me go blind?" I was willing to accept a little less treatment, a little more risk, to keep my eyesight.

After many, many discussions, my radiation oncologist and I agreed on a plan of 33 low-dose radiation treatments, which would reduce the likelihood of blindness. This was possible because the chemotherapy had been so effective. My doctor was upfront though. He said, "I can never take the risk of blindness lower than 15%. I can't radiate that area and promise that you won't lose your eyesight."

Thankfully, I didn't go blind. I've had no vision changes at all; ten years later, my vision is still 20/20. Honestly, I sometimes feel a bit embarrassed that I was so worried about it—I know blind people who have very fulfilling lives—but it was something I couldn't accept at the time of treatment.

I do not have a sense of smell...except for Windex and pine. So I can smell Windex and Christmas trees, but I'll never smell New York City garbage again. I do have a tendency toward dry mouth, but that has gotten much better over time. As a result, I got the first cavity of my life after cancer treatment and have to pay closer attention to my oral hygiene. Surprisingly, my pituitary function is still normal, and so are my thyroid and adrenal functions. I was able to get pregnant without assistance twice, and I had healthy pregnancies with fairly straightforward births. I've been able to breastfeed. At times, it feels very strange to have dodged what felt at the time to be a huge bullet—or many small bullets.

During radiation, I adopted a lot of "magical thinking." I would be lying there, wearing the mask they attach to the treatment table, thinking, *Just let the radiation touch what it needs to touch, and leave my eyes alone.* Or I'd think, *Breathe the toxin away from your optic nerves, away from your pituitary gland.* I had a friend who was very into guided imagery, and she gave me exercises to do during treatments and at home. At the time, it helped me control my nerves, in a situation over which I didn't have much control. Now that I'm so far away from it, I think that was the biggest benefit. I don't actually believe that all those exercises prevented blindness or preserved my pituitary function. When I think about it all now, I remember my mother telling me, "Control and the illusion of control are almost the same thing. We have no control. We can do our best, but we ultimately may not get the outcome we want."

Then came the process of recovering from cancer. It was a lot slower than I'd thought it would be. During treatment, I felt quite brave. But as I emerged from the physical trauma—when my hair started to grow back, my eyebrows and my eyelashes, all of that kind of stuff—I began to have moments of fear when I thought, *I can't believe I just got through that.*

The first three years were especially hard, with many peaks and valleys, because that's when you have the highest likelihood of recurrence. I kept thinking, *Will this next scan be the one to find a cluster of cancer cells?* The scan three years post treatment felt very ominous, because they told me that there was a high likelihood of recurrence in the third year, in the lungs. As I said, my mother had a recurrence in her lungs three years after breast cancer treatment, so there was a lot of anxiety at that scan. But it was also the scan that made me feel removed enough from the diagnosis to try and have a baby.

Five years after cancer treatment, I was still recovering physically, especially from fatigue. Little by little, that exhaustion lifted, but it took years for me to regain the energy that radiation sucked away. On the outside, I had long hair again, and I was healthy, active, and working. I had a healthy baby. But I was still recovering. Other people might not have seen it, but I could definitely feel it.

Now it's been 10 years. Sometimes it feels like I never had cancer, and sometimes it feels like it's Damocles' sword that could hit at any moment. Recently, I decided to do all of the genetic testing for cancer genes. For a long time I didn't feel like I needed the information, since I knew I wouldn't do a prophylactic mastectomy because I wanted to breastfeed. But then at some point, I was thinking about my kids. I felt if there's anything I could do to potentially minimize risk, I'd do it. A body can only take so much radiation. So I did the tests, and they all came back negative. I don't have a BRCA mutation or any of the other 10 or so genetic issues they can test for right now.

Cancer is a strange thing. There are days when I feel like maybe I should be a little more grateful that I'm alive. I still get annoyed with my kids, bored with my job. I don't feel grateful every day. When people say, "Cancer was a gift," I'm like, "What are you talking about?" It's an experience, for sure. It shaped me. I can never be quite the same. But I wouldn't say that I've come through the experience feeling every day like, "Wow, I feel so much happier about life!"

Actually, I might have felt the most joyful *during* my cancer treatment. My attitude was, "Well, if I die, I'd better die happy." So I dumped a lot of the "healthy living" that I was using as a shield against cancer and decided, "I'm going to get through cancer treatment doing what makes me happy." I thought about what made me happiest as a kid. That was watching the *Muppet* movies, eating buttered toast, and drinking as much hot chocolate as I could. So that's what I did, and I never went back. I would say I am healthy now—I eat well and exercise—but I feel much more open to living. Joyful? I'm dealing with the day-to-day. I'm sleep-deprived and caring for two small people under five. Maybe I'll feel more joyful when they're older.

Building Community, Changing Lives

Name: Lauren Chiarello Mika

Town: Ridgefield, CT

Diagnosis: Hodgkin's lymphoma; stage 2

Age at diagnosis: 23

Age now: 35

When an ENT told me the lump I felt on my collarbone might be lymphoma, it took me a second to register that lymphoma was cancer. I was actually by myself that day, but when I came back to meet with the head-and-neck surgeon, I brought my mom. From there, a tissue biopsy confirmed that I had stage 2A Hodgkin's lymphoma (HL). Luckily, Hodgkin's is one of the most curable types of cancers.

When I was diagnosed, I was just a year and a half out of college. I had recently moved to New York City, into an apartment on the Upper East Side with two roommates. I worked in special events and fundraising for an organization called Lenox Hill Neighborhood House, a social-services agency. I was energized to start my career, transitioning from the volunteer work I had done at Villanova University: Creating and managing fundraising events, raising awareness of various issues, and cultivating a community of supporters around them. I loved my work.

BEST ADVICE: Document your day-to-day—how you feel, what treatments you received, what doctor you saw. Writing down the basics was helpful, particularly when I was in the hospital. I had trouble remembering my day-to-day, in part because of high fevers. Because I wrote everything down, I always had the information. It empowered me. It's also a way to help stay in the moment, which is my other best advice: Take everything step by step.

Treatment was six months of chemotherapy, during which I worked full time. It was 12 treatments total, administered every other week. During the time that I was being treated, some friends decided to join Team in Training for the Leukemia and Lymphoma Society, to run the fall Nike Women's Marathon in San Francisco. They had never run a marathon but said, "We're taking on this challenge in your honor, in celebration of you and your strength."

Their experience motivated me to sign up for my first half marathon with Team in Training, just after I was declared in remission in summer 2008. Before, I had been a casual runner; I might do three miles and call it a

153

day. All that fall, I trained. I made a career move as well: I started working at Memorial Sloan Kettering Cancer Center, in the development office in fund-raising and event planning. I interviewed in my wig and never said anything about my diagnosis. I wanted to be hired for me, and I was.

Quickly it was race time, and I flew down to Florida. I didn't go alone—15 people came down to cheer me on for that weekend. Finishing the race that day, with so many loved ones cheering for me, was such an incredible and empowering experience. It was my first real understanding that community and connection are the pillars that carry us through life. That feeling has stayed with me through the last nine years.

Maybe the revelation wouldn't have been so monumental, except that my cancer journey didn't end there. During the race weekend, I felt a lump above my collarbone, in exactly the same place as before. Pretty wild, because having a recurrence with HL is uncommon. I was surprised. Actually, I was devastated. I was 24. All I wanted was to be out, doing the things my friends were doing, exploring and living. I felt completely sidelined. And my first treatment was nothing compared to what I ended up going through the second time.

Before starting my second treatment—which I did at Memorial Sloan Kettering—I froze my eggs. The first time I went through chemo, the medical team wasn't concerned about infertility. This time they warned me that it could be a real issue. Luckily there was an organization called Fertile Hope, now acquired by Livestrong, which funded what would have been an expensive fertility-preservation process. I had to give myself hormone shots to build up my egg production. The fertility team retrieved and froze 24 eggs, which they told me was an amazing outcome. Ever since, I've paid $1000 a year in storage fees.

With that done, I had to leave work for six months to go through treatment. There were two preconditioning chemotherapy treatments. From there, I had a scan to see how the cancer looked. The scan was nearly clear, so at that point I was ready to collect my own stem cells and prepare for an autologous stem cell transplant. Shortly after, I had two weeks of radiation, high-dose chemotherapy, and then the stem cell transplant. The cancer was not in my bone marrow, so I was able to have my own stem cells transplanted. Man, that just rocked me. Essentially, stem cell therapy works this way: They give you such high-dose chemo that it takes you to the brink of death. Your blood counts are zero, and then they infuse you with your own stem cells to rescue you.

I struggled with high fevers and sores. I was in the hospital, in isolation, for six weeks. Taking a shower was the victory for the day. It hurt to swallow my own saliva. I could barely eat—I ate mushed-up pancakes for a month and not much else. From there I went home to my parents in Westchester County. My first nephew was born just three days after I got out of the hospital. We got stronger together that summer. In 2019, he turned 10.

I went back to work at Memorial Sloan Kettering in August, was there for three years, then moved on to Helen Keller International, a global-health organization. At Memorial Sloan Kettering, I continued to participate in team fundraising efforts—Fred's Team and Cycle for Survival. With Fred's Team, I ran two full marathons. My commitment to Cycle for Survival continues today. Each year I have a five-bike, 20-person team. This year we raised over $25,000.

I also fundraised for First Descents. In 2010, I went white-water kayaking in Vail, Colorado, for a week with 14 other young-adult cancer survivors. First Descents provides the week of adventure therapy completely free. It was an incredible opportunity to connect with other people who went through something similar and can relate. It's a really beautiful way to create connection and community and to understand that you're not alone.

In 2012, the New York City Marathon was canceled due to Hurricane Sandy. So a few fellow Fred's Team members headed with me to Harrisburg, Pennsylvania, and I completed my first marathon. What's unique about Fred's Team is that you can allocate your funds to any area of cancer research that you want. I had mine dedicated to lymphoma and the survivorship program.

I was still determined to run the New York City Marathon, and I did it the following year. Just around mile 16 and a half, you run past Memorial Sloan Kettering, on First Avenue. You're greeted with giant balloon arches. The hospital brings down patients from the pediatric department to cheer you on. Words can't describe the energy there, running past that building. I wanted to run past the place that saved my life—and I did, in 2013.

A year after my transplant, a friend took me to a barre class, and I fell in love with the method. It's a full-body core-strength and conditioning class. You use your own body weight to build strength, flexibility, and mobility through targeted movements. Initially, I found the method helpful in increasing my running pace. But after five years as a student, I started wondering: *Could I teach?*

I didn't know if I could—if I'd be good at it or even like it. But I pushed past the resistance and signed up for Exhale's 40-hour teacher training. I wasn't very good when I started. No one is. One of my favorite phrases is, "Every expert was once a novice." To progress in anything and hone a skill, you have to practice. It was not easy—very humbling. It helped me build self-confidence. Becoming a teacher helped me discover the person I was meant to be: Someone who shares her passions with her students. My mission is to hold space for them and inspire them to get stronger, in both body and mind.

Four years later, I'm still teaching barre—and now Pilates and TRX as well. I left my full-time job in 2014 and combined teaching with freelance event planning, working with nonprofits and startups. One year in, I was making more than I had in my last full-time salaried position. Nearly all of my work comes through word of mouth; I feel so grateful for that. I put my heart and soul into everything I do.

This past year I've added corporate wellness programming to my business. I teach classes and also curate panels and workshops around specific themes. I partner with the amazing humans I've met over these last few years in the health and wellness space. I remember sitting at a desk for eight, nine, ten, or eleven hours a day and feeling like Humpty Dumpty sitting on the wall—quite sedentary throughout the day. When I go into companies, I create a session that's both restorative and energizing. I make class fun, but I really teach to educate. I like to see the progress in my students over time. It's really why I do what I do.

People go through so many different life hurdles. I happened to experience cancer. I know many people who went through cancer and who are not here anymore. I truly feel a calling to share my story, which is one of resilience and bouncing back. We have the power to change our lives at any given moment, on any given day. I deeply believe that. Our days are made up of choices and habits, and we have the ability to make positive change.

For me, I deepened my relationship with exercise. I was an active person, but now exercise and movement are ingrained in each day. Don't get me wrong, I have my rest days! I have a better understanding of the connection between body and mind. When we move, we really do feel better. Exercise releases amazing hormones. Our brain is happier.

We're living in a challenging time on a lot of different levels, but I feel like there's so much good to be done. My greatest joy is being able to live life every day and share my passion with others. I love meeting new people and hearing their stories. I love helping people, and making introductions when missions and passions align.

I continue to share my health journey on my blog, www.ChiChiLifeNYC.com, and on Instagram: @chichilifenyc. Health struggles don't stop when you're a cancer survivor; they're a part of life. I speak regularly at Memorial Sloan Kettering's nurse orientation about my experience as a young-adult cancer patient. The audiences are 50 to 100 people who are starting a new role in the nursing space at the hospital. I share how open communication was critical to my care. I felt like I was supported and I could ask any question. No matter who walked in the door, I was cared for on many levels.

Speaking is how I give back. It was so helpful for me to connect with others who had been through cancer. I want to honor the people who helped me. I had a fellow teacher tell me just the other day how she appreciated my blog and community. "I had open-heart surgery two years ago, and no one really knows," she confided. I was so blown away by her courage to share. It was a reminder to me that whatever discomfort or anxiety I might have about standing on a stage or sharing my story is worth it if I can have a positive impact on even one person.

Finding a Voice with C.D.R.E.A.M.

· ·

Name: Tiffany Dyba

Town: New York, New York

Diagnosis: Breast cancer; stage 1; invasive ductal carcinoma

Age at diagnosis: 35

Age now: 37

When I think about how much my life has changed recently, the story starts a year before my cancer diagnosis. In January 2017, I got a big promotion at work. Instead of being happy with what I had worked for years to achieve, I sobbed on the train home and then on my 10-minute walk to my apartment in Astoria, Queens. To the friends I had grown up with in Ohio, I was living the dream: working in Manhattan, leading the recruitment team at Burberry after years at Tiffany & Co. I love fashion—but after working in jobs related to it for 15 years, I felt like I had turned into someone who was constantly keeping up with the Joneses. I was starting to feel like my outside didn't match my inside.

2017 became my year of discovery. I started working with a career coach, and after interviewing at a lot of places that still didn't feel like the right fit, I decided to put my recruitment experience to work helping others make career transitions.

BEST ADVICE: Don't be ashamed to go through the emotional curve. Nothing is off the table. You're allowed to feel whatever you want to feel.

When I told Burberry what I was up to in July, they suggested that I stay on part time while I got my new coaching business up and running.

At the start of 2018, I vacationed in Iceland with my husband. That's when I first felt the lump in my breast, while I was taking a shower. Two weeks after we got home, my doctor sent me for a mammogram and ultrasound—and instead of letting me go, they asked me to wait for a radiologist to review it. I knew that was a bad sign. A week later, I had a biopsy, and the Friday after, I was running on the treadmill when the official call came that I had cancer. That was March 8th. Two weeks later, I had a double mastectomy. The cancer was only in my left breast, but my feeling was, "While you're in there, just do it."

March 8th was also the day I wrote my first blog post, although I didn't publish it until later. I called it C.D.R.E.A.M, which is Cancer Doesn't Rule Everything Around Me—a play on Wu Tang, because I love hip-hop. The blog's URL is tiffversuscancer.com, and I started an Instagram at the same time. All of my posts, with the exception of maybe one or two, I wrote in real time at different points in my journey, because I wanted my audience to read real emotion. Evernote is my best friend. If I'm in the park and I'm upset about something, I'll pull out my phone and jot a paragraph down. I'm very much that "in the moment" kind of writer. If I'm crying, I need to write about it then, because it makes the writing better.

My surgery was on the 29th of March. So many people told me that I should have someone with me the first time I looked at my post-mastectomy body. So I did, and was I was bracing for a crime scene. But I wasn't upset at all. My expanders were in, so there was already something there. There was a big scar, but I thought, *This isn't so bad. I can work with this. When the implants go in and I get a nipple tattoo, I'll clean up real nice.*

My plastic surgeon had prepared me well. He showed me a lot of before-and-after pictures, so I knew what to expect. I've never had a really intense connection to my boobs. I will tell you other people in my life have. I grew up tall and lanky and was always flat-chested, and then somehow, junior year, all of a sudden I had double-D boobs, and people thought I had a boob job in high school. I was like, no, guys, I really didn't. They've gotten me out of a few speeding tickets, but I've never been particularly attached to having big boobs.

I've been married for 10 years, so he's stuck with me and my crime-scene boobs now. If I were out there dating I'd probably feel different, because that could be tough. Even for me, there was a little bit of insecurity at first. Having sex the first couple of times, I wanted to leave my shirt on. My husband was like, "Take it off, girl." That helped me go from "I look like an alien" to "Let's just do this." It took me a few times to feel feminine. I guess I also figured that if I wasn't going to be sexually stimulated by my boobs anymore, then what was the point of taking my shirt off? I got in my own head a few times and couldn't let myself be present during sex. Add that to the diminished libido you have during chemo, and you are really not having a wild Saturday night. This too shall pass, right?

Writing had always been in the backdrop of what I do—but now it's in the forefront. That started during my year of discovery, when I was blogging for my new business every week. Sharing my knowledge with people gets me excited. When I was diagnosed, I was scouring the internet looking for resources and women under 40, and I couldn't really find any. That's a problem, because there are so many people getting diagnosed with breast cancer and cancer in general under 40. I knew immediately that I wanted to share my experience in a blog, to start to fill that hole. I also knew that writing itself, the process, would be cathartic, as it has been my whole life.

When I started C.D.R.E.A.M., I didn't care if it reached 200 people or 20 million. I just hoped anyone who truly needed it would find it and get help, with a little humor thrown in. Call it denial, call it insensitivity, but my feeling is that if you can't laugh about it, you might as well be dead.

When I was diagnosed, I had already started the process of getting clearer on my priorities. That has continued. I look at friendships differently now. I used to have so many acquaintances. I felt like I was always running, trying to do everything. Now I'm really comfortable just spending time with a few people who really understand me and add value to my life. I'm also prioritizing my health now. I'm a vegetarian and borderline vegan. I'm drinking a lot less—I have to. Not that I drank a ton before, but I like my wine. Now I'm so much more mindful of my body and my mind. I pushed that kind of thing to the side before, because I never thought that cancer would happen to me.

Cancer has given me more of a voice and purpose. I had a therapist who told me she thought I had a personality type that was meant to play big. That resonated, but I felt like I wanted the "big" to be about a purpose bigger than me. So I started the business, hoping to help women who are feeling stuck in their career. It's interesting that, after my diagnosis, I'm helping women who are stuck in a different way, looking for support and real information about cancer. I was literally on the table, getting ready to be put under for my double mastectomy, thinking, *I can't die, because people need me. I need to help people.* Not self-aggrandizing, like in a Kanye West way—I just know that cancer has given me the confidence to execute a lot of things I would otherwise have been afraid to do.

How We Talk About Cancer Matters

Name: Emily Garnett

Town: Mount Kisco, New York

Diagnosis: Breast cancer; stage 4; ER+; invasive ductal carcinoma with metastases to bones, brain, liver, and lung

Age at diagnosis: 32

Age now: 34

As I sit down to edit this essay created from my interview, I realize that it has been a full year since these words took life. An entire year of living with metastatic breast cancer, an entire year of change and growth, and an entire year that has brought me closer to my eventual death. I want to use these words, both then and now, to recognize the shifts that took place, in language, advocacy, and understanding of my life with metastatic breast cancer.

In the early months of my diagnosis, I found that people only talk about breast cancer in very hushed tones. Even family members and close friends were hesitant to utter the word "cancer" and instead preferred to talk about my "situation" or "illness." We need to recognize the importance of language as a vessel of control. If one in eight of us is going to get breast cancer in our lifetime, it's not something we should be talking about in such a hush-hush way. How do we talk about metastatic breast cancer?

> BEST ADVICE: (received and given): I need to allow myself to be sad. I mean really, gut-wrenchingly, eyes-blurred-from-tears, can't-stop-sobbing, can't-get-out-of-bed sad. I need to let myself continue to grieve, to feel—to recognize that, despite being able to push through a lot of this stuff, I am navigating an ongoing trauma, one that truly, truly sucks. It really does, and it doesn't get better. My new normal shifts and changes, and, to an extent, I can adapt to that; but I can't run away from it, and I can't ignore it.

Language can offer autonomy in situations—such as life with a cancer diagnosis—in which little other control can be offered. We exist in a point in time where cancer therapies are developing at a rapid and exciting pace. We see immunotherapies being developed and tested with surprising and encouraging results. These results certainly drive our utilization of language, but to what end?

Metastatic breast cancer is, I believe, the second-most deadly cancer for women. It kills 116 people a day. Now, that's a shocking statistic. But how can we classify ourselves in a way that is both empowering and informative?

Are we terminal, often with less than one year to live? Yes, some of us are. Others of us are veering into the territory of chronic disease, with years and years of life lived showing no evidence of disease—yet the specter of progression never leaves. Are we incurable? Initial immunotherapy studies are indicating that, in some individualized cases, breast cancer can be eradicated from the body. Yet, we return to this number—116 people a day. This number is growing, and it encompasses all of these terms and other ones too, such as "thriver."

I prefer the most direct language: I am living with metastatic breast cancer. I will likely not beat this cancer, but I refuse to concede the breaths afforded to me at this singular moment in time.

The language we use to talk about our disease can be tremendously personal. A year ago, I was taking Lupron, Letrozole, and my sixth cycle of Ibrance, which is a targeted therapy. The treatment itself was not too bad, not so virulently toxic as chemo. I never lost my hair. I went in once a month for Lupron injections, which put me into chemical menopause. I'm permanently infertile and can never have any more children. My first PET scan showed that the medication was working and that there was a decently good decrease in metabolic activity in all of my tumors, and some of them looked like they had resolved completely. Everyone, myself included, was very cautiously hopeful that this could be a drug I could be on long-term. My oncologist said, "Until we have reason to think otherwise—and we don't—it could be many, many years."

And then that narrative changed. Approximately one year after starting the targeted-therapy treatment, we discovered it had stopped working. It had failed—or my body had failed, which is how I felt in the weeks following the news. "Many, many years" turned into "months to years." The illness I had hoped to manage as chronic turned into a more acute, challenging game of leap-frog. I began a clinical trial, and after two months on the study drug, once again I showed stable scans. I had close to no side effects and was reclaiming, once again, pieces of my life that had drifted into the ether.

Then I started noticing some unusual headaches, some dizziness. My oncologist ordered a brain MRI, which revealed two small lesions in my parietal lobe. I underwent stereotactic radiosurgery (targeted brain radiation) to eliminate both lesions and was able to continue on the trial for another month. However, new symptoms called for another set of scans, and we discovered further sites of disease in my liver and, potentially, my left lung. I am currently off the clinical trial and exploring additional treatment options.

On January 1, 2018, I made an unusual New Year's resolution (for me). Instead of pledging to save money, lose weight, exercise more, or find a new hobby, I pledged to myself that I would live fearlessly. I pledged to live in a way that removes excuses to avoid doing the things I've previously been afraid of doing, or waiting for the right time to do them. For me, the right time is now. Entering 2019, that pressure mounted, as I felt the push internally that I was "on the clock" more than ever. I'm reaching out to people saying,

"Look, I want to talk to you. I like what you're doing. I want to be part of it. I want to have these dialogues about what's going on and what you think about it."

I've said that life with metastatic breast cancer is the worst club with the best people. Truthfully, I've never been around so many women and men who were so driven and on fire with passion—about finding treatments, raising money, and addressing the need for more knowledge and, ultimately, cures. I am starting to understand my role within this larger community and create a space for that role. Through that, I have discovered and created a support system that I didn't previously have.

I would be fully lying if I said the dynamic nature of my illness wasn't terrifying. In recent days, particularly since the discovery of liver involvement, I have often felt overcome by wave after wave of bad news, unable to surface to catch my breath. A year ago, I talked, somewhat brazenly, about how metastatic illness was inappropriately termed as terminal. I had the good sense to differentiate it from chronic disease, as well, because it truly does limit one's life expectancy. But I said, a year ago, that metastatic disease is incurable but treatable. That it is not a chronic disease, necessarily, like diabetes—because a chronic disease by definition indicates that someone is going to live with that disease without a reduced life expectancy, which is not the case with metastatic breast cancer. The average life expectancy is about 29 months. That's the mean, not the median, so it's a statistic that doesn't capture the full picture—but it is a sobering statistic. I began to relabel my disease as a serious illness that fell between the two spaces of chronic and terminal. This gave me a modicum of empowerment over my uncontrollable situation.

Yet the spectre still loomed. My treatments were becoming less effective, and I began to recognize the limitations of our collective body of knowledge about my illness—both my personal nuances that allow the cancer cells to evade treatment, and the nuances of research attention and dollars. I am staring down the lens of a different gun these days. This gun looms much bigger.

You may be wondering how I handle the fear that comes with living with metastatic breast cancer. I'm being a little glib here, but also truthful: I have a very, very good psychiatrist. I had a predisposition for depression and anxiety prior to this diagnosis, and I had some untreated postpartum depression and anxiety. So I knew that I was very much going into the belly of the beast. Within a couple of days of my diagnosis, I called my primary-care doctor and said, "I need you to recommend the best psychiatrist that you know, who has experience working with cancer patients and is going to help me manage this from a mental-health standpoint."

I began working with a wonderful psychiatrist. She and I tweaked a good combination of antidepressants—which also helped with a lot of the menopausal hot flashes, strangely enough. She prescribed antianxiety medications to help me sleep. I knew that I needed to be ahead of whatever storm was coming for me, and this proactive mission of self-care has continued to serve me well. I refuse to let myself suffer needlessly.

Every night, right before I go to bed, I take my Ativan and my Tylenol PM, or melatonin, Ambien, or Oxycodone (if my pain levels demand it), and then I take a really hot shower for about 15 minutes. Before my medications kick in, I let myself go to those really difficult, dark places. I ask myself questions like, "If I know I'm going to die, what do I want to have in place? How do I want to structure my legacy? What things do I want to leave my husband and son? What information, what pieces of myself?" Then I get out of the shower and I make some notes, including related things I'll work on during the day. I have a little folder on my laptop that I keep all those notes in. I do as much as I can stomach, knowing that within 10 or 15 minutes that medication is going kick in, and it's really going to help me sleep. Honestly, I know it sounds weird to do it before bed, but I sleep better that way, knowing that I have exorcized that demon for the day.

If I don't let myself go to those dark places, that awful rage, that bottomless sadness bottlenecks and bubbles up to the surface at times when I'm uncomfortable with it, and it becomes far less productive. By doing this, I start to feel like I have a measure of control over the worst situation I can imagine, which would be passing away without having lived a life that I feel is good, and full, and settled.

I have so much joy in my life. I'm sitting at my computer at my desk with my cat, and we're looking out into our backyard. And I have a window open, and the window is perfect. It's gorgeous outside and green and adorable. A family of deer often comes around right before sunset. There's a little cardinal who appears. This little cardinal has been kind of a spirit guide for me in this whole process of reclaiming my life—the life that we never would have chosen, but the life we have anyway.

I spent a lot of time after my diagnosis really hashing out questions: What kind of life do I want to live? What kind of day do I want to have? What makes my cup feel full, and what makes me go to bed feeling fulfilled or feeling like I'm living a good life? I like writing, I like drinking coffee, I like working out and playing with my son—taking him to the farm, and to go berry picking, and to the park. Finding the little moments in cooking dinner with him. Finding the little moments that give you the opportunity to appreciate day-to-day life. It's trite and also so fundamental, because it's the softness that gives us the space to find strength.

Before I go to sleep, I peek into my son's room and see him all snuggled up in his bed, and I think of all his milestones that I have been a part of in the last year and a half. The start of preschool, moving from a crib to a big-kid bed, potty training, and his development from a toddler into a running, growing, talkative, serious, creative little boy. My son was two years old when I was diagnosed. These are such formative years, and I have to remind myself that instead of thinking of the length of time that I won't be physically available for him, I have to focus on the time we have now, to create the space for him to grow into the future.

The first few weeks after diagnosis, I kept asking myself, *Is this going to get better?* Now I think it's better to say, "No, it's not going to get better." Saying that is really empowering, because it gives you a construct to build from. This is the new normal. It's not better—it's scary, it's awful, and you're completely justified to feel all the feelings, to mourn and be angry, to be sad and to bottom out. And then, slowly, you begin to create a new life, a new understanding of what your existence looks like through the lens of this disease. The life you never chose. You pull from the depths of your soul, to create space for light in a situation that is so unbelievably difficult.

Art to Heal the Spirit

Name: Robin Glazer

Town: New York City, NY

Diagnosis: Breast cancer; stage 1, then stage 4; ER+

Age at diagnosis: 37, then 53

Age now: 63

I helped to found an organization called the Creative Center back in 1994, after I'd finished a year of treatment for breast cancer. I had 52 chemo sessions, taking drugs that are not used too often anymore—a combination called CMFVP. We founded the Creative Center on the belief that "medicine cures the body, but art heals the spirit." It was based on both my personal experience and the experience of the two other founders—one of whom, Adrienne Assail, died soon after we began. Geraldine Herbert, the first director, retired in 2006. As for me, I was rediagnosed in 2009, and I'm now going into year 10 of my stage 4 diagnosis with no evidence of disease. At 63, I am now the organization's director, though we merged with University Settlement in 2011 and are no longer an independent nonprofit.

BEST ADVICE: It came from my former oncologist, an orthodox Jewish doctor. First he said it in Hebrew, then he said it in Yiddish, and then he said it in English: "You know when God closes one door, he opens another." And then, of course, months later, when I told him all the things I was now doing, he said, "But I didn't tell you to go through every door!"

When I was diagnosed the first time, I was a young mom of five children. I had started my family when I was just 23 and had my children in fairly quick succession. I was always a really creative person, but I hadn't done my own work since before I had kids. Initially, I was a dancer; I turned to visual art when I became an art teacher in schools. At that time, my artwork was always in the service of others. We always had fabulous birthday parties and great Halloween costumes. My kids had amazing murals in their bedrooms.

During my year of treatment, I had to take a three-hour bus trip every week, from where we had moved in Pennsylvania back to New York, where I chose to have treatment. Those trips became time spent reconnecting with myself. I started talking to artists and survivors, plus reconnecting with old friends, and it inspired me to start working on my own art again. I started sketching myself. I had what was then known as a "radical mastectomy," to remove one breast. I wasn't offered reconstruction, but I wasn't disturbed by how I was going to look. I started looking for images of women with mastectomies, but there was almost nothing out there. And so I did a self-portrait two days before surgery, and then one several weeks after, after the surgical drains were removed, with my one breast. I did these drawings looking in a tiny makeup mirror, because I didn't have a full one. Can you imagine? One little section at a time—but I think looking at myself in little sections was probably an easier way of seeing my new body all at once.

So that was my foray into thinking about my *self*—these paintings of the physical self. Almost immediately, the paintings and drawings began to go from highly realistic to almost phantasmagoric, placing my naked self with one breast into a variety of settings. It felt very freeing. Could I see myself in Tahiti? Yes, I could. Did I feel like I was underground climbing through a minefield, or in a coal mine? Absolutely. Did I see myself with a magician's sword going through my neck? Yes, I did. Some of these self-portraits were clothed and some were not clothed, because I realized that losing my breast was not the issue for me. The issue was facing death.

I had a show of my self-portraits. Afterward, the local reporter's news headline was, "From Selfless to Selfish." He told me that he had written "self-full" but that the typesetters thought that was a mistake and altered it to selfish! So I actually have that in a little frame, and I think it's perfect. Cancer gave me permission to be selfish!

The beauty of a serious illness is that you're given permission to take the time to explore yourself. None of us know how much time we have. None of us know what's going to happen next. But people with cancer understand better than the rest of the world that our time is limited. You can take advantage of that and say, "Hopefully I'll get the rest of my life, but I may not. What am I going to do with the time I have? Who do I want to be?" Many healthy people, even very old ones, fail to face the reality of their own death. To me, they're missing an opportunity.

Just yesterday I visited one of the Creative Center's Hospital Artists-in-Residence who works in oncology. She was sitting with a woman who was getting chemotherapy, and the woman was surrounded by a gallery of small paintings that she had done—some created with the artist while this woman was there for treatment every three weeks, others created as "homework" between chemos. The Artist-in-Residence would give her visual prompts to work from. The woman was in her late 60s or early 70s and had never painted in her life before our program.

As we were chatting, I noticed one of her arms had swollen up. She was constantly rotating her hand around, as if it was bothering her. When she saw me looking at it, she said, "Oh, never mind, it's just pain." Here she was, chemo drugs dripping into her, wrist killing her, and yet all of that she pushed aside, because she really wanted to engage around her artworks—what did I think about them, how could she improve them? She was so excited. Matisse is one of her favorite artists, she told me, and she talked about color. For the first time in many years, color came back into her life after her diagnosis, because she had an opportunity to take time to notice it.

She went on about what our art program had done for her. Then she corrected herself—she said it was cancer that had made her an artist, because it had given her the opportunity to slow down and truly look, then to change what she saw through her eyes into what she saw in her soul. Slowing down—that's the gift that illness offers you.

In 26 years of working at the Creative Center, I've worked with thousands of people—some very intimately through our hospital program, where I get to sit with the artists we've hired and talk to the patients one-on-one as they're creating art. When we first started, in the mid '90s, we only worked with women, because they were very underserved in terms of complementary programs; but now we also work with men. Again and again, I see how art helps transform a time of illness into an incredible blossoming of the self.

Another woman had breast cancer, and she worked all through her initial diagnosis and treatment. Then, when it metastasized, she felt fine but decided to "take advantage of being sick," as she put it. She went on disability and decided to explore silk painting, which she had learned in our program. She became an amazing silk painter and did some incredible work that was not very traditional. She spent the last few years of her life doing something that she didn't even know she could do, and loving every minute.

Right now there's a participant who has been working with us for about two years. She had never done art of any kind before. She started to take all different types of classes with us—writing, puppetry, painting. Then she called one day and said, "I have the audacity to apply for a

BEST ADVICE: Cancer: use it or lose it. Move forward as though every day may be your last and keep stringing those together for your lifetime – whatever that is.

scholarship for a residency in watercolor at a craft school in North Carolina, a folk-art school. Would you write me a recommendation?" How could I say no? I don't even really know what her artwork looks like. But here was a person who saw her own opportunity and decided to seize it! She had once struck me as a woman who had never been able to find herself. She is a New Yorker, alone, as are many of our participants. That's great while you're working, but when you're not working, it's not so great. You lose your coworkers, you lose that community where you've spent so many hours each day, year after year. Now she's connected to other people in our program, and I see her at various art venues, places that were never part of her life before cancer.

Another participant is a woman in her 80s who was an attorney all her working life. Fabulous dresser—but the crankiest person you've ever met. She has lived in the same apartment for 60 years. She came to New York as a "career girl" but now spends her entire life creating art—she learned how to do all of that with us after cancer. Because she can be cantankerous, I think people in her former life have kept distance from her. Somehow, though, in these art workshops, with some encouragement, her soft and gentle side comes out. And other people are connecting with her. She rides home with them. We got a call yesterday from a woman and I said, "How did you hear about us?" And she said, "There's this woman on the bus..." And it was her, chatting with strangers on the bus. It turned out the woman she referred didn't even have cancer—she hadn't mentioned it was a prerequisite!

There are many, many, many stories. Sitting on my desk right now is a book of essays and poetry written by somebody who took creative writing classes and self-published a book. She's never written a word before in her life!

I was talking to a group of oncology fellows about my own story, and one of them looked at me and said, "You almost seem happy to have had cancer." And I said, "Actually, I'm just happy, and then I had cancer." When I was diagnosed, someone I knew told someone else I knew that I had become "the cancer queen." When I heard that, I said, "OK, great! I'll take it. I don't want to become the cancer victim—that's worse." I want everybody to dance through cancer, eat through cancer, paint through cancer. It's about discovering yourself and all the things you can do, instead of thinking you have to live your life for someone else. Not to sound New Age-y or spiritual, because I'm not, but you can become your true self after diagnosis, whatever that is. You just have to give yourself permission to let that in. Cancer gives you permission to take risks! Be the queen you always knew you were—or wanted to be!

Now, at 63, I'm a grandmother of very young children. In a very short time I'm going to have four grandchildren under the age of three. When I'm in full, active "grandma mode," there's no part of me that is thinking about whatever I'm going through physically, emotionally, or work-wise. All of that gets pushed out of the way and I'm 100% in as their grandmother. It's another way of being self-full, because you look at these kids and you realize they're so much a part of you—biologically but also creatively. It's like a full expression of love in something that you create. That's what art can be, too.

Healing in Heels

Name: Yoko Katz

Location: Westchester County, New York

Diagnosis: Breast cancer; ER+, PR+, HER2+ ("triple positive")

Age at diagnosis: 36

Age now: 41

When I was diagnosed with breast cancer, I was married, and our son was 8 years old. I was a Ph.D student in economics; I was writing my dissertation on industrial organization of the fashion industry. It was almost done, and I was working as an adjunct lecturer at the Fashion Institute of Technology. I was teaching three courses per semester.

At the time, I considered myself one of the healthiest people in the neighborhood. I ran regularly—five, six times a week, 20 to 40 minutes a run. I grew my own vegetables during the summer, totally organic. I went to a farmer's market when possible. I bought organic food. And I was juicing every single day in the morning, with kale, apples, orange, lemon, and some other vegetables. I had no family history of breast cancer.

BEST ADVICE: One day before my mastectomy, I requested an emergency meeting with my doctor. I wasn't sure that I wanted to have a single mastectomy instead of a double. Even though I wasn't positive for BRCA mutations, wasn't it better to be worry-free? I really appreciate what my doctor said. He told me that I seemed to be worrying that one part of my body, which is still healthy, could have possible future cancer. Then he told me this was true for any of my healthy organs. Would I want to get rid of all of them? So that gave me the answer. I kept my healthy breast.

One day in the shower, I found a lump. I thought it might be related to my period. I didn't pay too much attention, because I considered myself a very healthy person. I let it sit for another couple weeks, but I still felt it. It wasn't really changing, even though I had had my period.

So I started thinking, *Oh. Maybe it's something. I don't know.* I asked my husband if he could feel it. And he said, "Yeah. There is something." It was about the size of a large pea. My husband said I should check it out, but I still let it sit. That's how much I didn't feel that I had cancer.

One day I started getting back to work on my dissertation. My husband stopped by my desk and said, "So, did you make an appointment?"

And I said, "What appointment?"

Finally, I made the appointment. From there on things went very quickly. I had a mammogram, then an ultrasound. Then I had to go back for a biopsy. I wasn't thinking it was going to be a big deal. I was grading exams, casually waiting for my turn. When it came, I walked in, and the biopsy turned out to involve a really big machine. I wasn't really ready for it. It was traumatic. I couldn't stand up afterward. I had driven myself to the hospital, but I had to call my friend to pick me up.

The week after the biopsy, I got a phone call from the radiologist, who said, "Hi. All three biopsy sites show cancer." I was in such a state of shock that I had no response. My husband was there, and he started crying. That's how I was diagnosed.

"So what's my next step?" I asked the radiologist. He told me I had to find a breast surgeon. I said, "How do I do that?" I had no idea! The place where I had the mammography turned out to have a group of breast surgeons working at the hospital. So I started from there. I was very anxious and took the first appointment I could get, four days later. The radiologist had said he wasn't in a position to tell me anything more than I had cancer. So I didn't know what stage or anything else. I had to wait. The days before the appointment were a nightmare to me. All the information I could find on the Internet was horrifying. The lump that had felt very small suddenly started feeling really big. The first thing that came to my mind was, *My son is only 8 years old.*

At first, the surgeon told me I had estrogen-receptor-positive and progesterone-receptor- positive breast cancer, which determined my treatment. I was stage 1. He told me two options. I could do a mastectomy, reconstruction, and tamoxifen, either with or without chemotherapy.

The two options were so different that I wasn't sure which one to pick. So I found a doctor for a second opinion, and he told me the exact same thing. At that point, I was confident that either choice was good—but which one was better? It was a big decision. Obviously, not going through chemo sounded fantastic—but at the same time, I didn't want to risk the future, so part of me said pick the chemotherapy. It was very difficult for somebody who'd only just learned she had breast cancer to choose one of them.

Meanwhile, what I didn't know was that they were still trying to identify whether the cancer was HER2 positive or negative. The next time I saw my surgeon, he told me there was good news and bad news. That bad news was that it was HER2 positive as well. The good news was that there were good medications to treat that—but the original options had to be changed. Now chemotherapy was definite. This new information made the decision for me. I didn't want to go to chemotherapy, but that's the path I had to take.

Quickly I learned that every breast surgeon, and every breast cancer patient, works with multiple doctors. I needed an oncologist and a plastic surgeon. I also learned that going through chemo could damage my ovaries. If I wanted to get pregnant in the future, which at that point I did, I was advised to preserve my eggs. So that was a fourth doctor. We really wanted to have another child—but working on my dissertation while raising one child, and trying to raise him bilingual, was a lot. I am the only one in my home who can speak Japanese, so I put in a lot of time speaking in the language with my son. We had been waiting until I finished my dissertation to have a second child.

After my surgery, I still had really long hair. Before doing chemo, I decided to donate it, and I contacted my hair stylist. She told me that she could help. So I cut my hair very short, which I really liked. Losing my hair later was sad, but I'm glad that I was able to donate it.

At the same time, I started seeing a fertility doctor. I learned I only had one chance to retrieve eggs before chemotherapy, and we didn't know how successful it would be. The doctor told us there was an alternative: to cut out my ovaries, freeze them, and then reconnect them after chemo. They could go right back on the job! Hearing that was very surreal. I was very seriously concerned, but still I had to laugh. I was like, "What? Never thought of that. This is very scientific." I made an appointment for that procedure, just in case, but luckily I was able to preserve 11 eggs and create embryos.

All this stress upon stress was right after my mastectomy. I had surgical tubes coming out of my sides, but I had to go into the city to see the fertility specialist—and also to a local facility to do blood tests every two days. All I wanted was to be in bed, recovering from the surgery, but I didn't have the luxury to do it. I had to get up and go to these next treatments. It was summer, so at least I didn't have to worry about teaching.

Then the chemotherapy started. I went 6 times, every three weeks. It was really hard. I lost my sense of taste almost completely. All food looked gray to me because there was no enjoyment in it. I was only eating because I had to eat. My mouth got sore, too, and the texture of food was not pleasant for me. I ate more soup than solid food.

Of course, the hair loss came. But it was expected, so I was ready to go. I bought my first wig in orange. I decided that if I had to do this, I would do it in my own way. The school year would begin again in September, and my first chemo was in mid August. I knew that hair loss was going to kick in right when I went back to teaching. I reduced my teaching load from three to two courses, both of which were based on my dissertation. No one could teach them but me. I wanted to look like the "me" from before cancer when I stood in front of students again. I wanted to be fashionable; I wanted to look professional. And so I put in an extra effort. Instead of thinking of a complete look as being from neck to toe, I started thinking of my fashion from head to toe. I had different wigs and hats to match to my outfits. I started buying scarves. It became more important to consider style as a whole, including my hairless head.

I started thinking about writing a blog soon after diagnosis, but I didn't have time to write at first. So many doctors' appointments, so much research to do, so many decisions to make. But once chemo started, I gave up a lot of things that I normally do, like taking care of my child and making meals. I let other people handle these for me. I did participate when I could. But I had more time to sit and write—and that's when I finally started my blog. I already knew that I was going to call it Heal in Heels, because that's the road I wanted to take.

When I learned that I would lose my hair, the only images I could find on the Internet were of very sick-looking cancer patients, wearing scarves in a way that made it clear they were "cancer scarves." I thought, *I can't go in front of my fashionable students with that look.* I wanted to be a little bit more creative. Since I'm in the fashion field, I thought that maybe I could propose to the world another way to approach this—so that women, and maybe even men, wouldn't have to feel miserable and pity themselves during these treatments. I wanted people to feel like they were still themselves during cancer treatment, with the help of fashion.

I didn't have to dress every single day. But when necessary, I could style myself so that when I went out in public, I still had privacy. People wouldn't give me looks that said, "Oh, pity that she has to go through treatment." I knew I was a cancer patient 24-7, but I didn't have to announce that to the public all the time. I really craved normality during treatment, because everything seems to be upside down.

The idea of making hats came to me when I was sitting in the waiting room to get chemo. When I had my scarves on, other patients would say, "Wow. How do you do that?" They wanted to know how to put themselves together. I started doing some demonstrations here and there, but a lot of people had difficulties doing it themselves. It took me a while to learn how to put on my scarves in a way that looks fabulous. It wasn't overnight. I did a lot of YouTubing and trial and error. But I had a gut feeling that I wanted to look OK—to look nice, even.

I started thinking that maybe I could make hats to help cancer patients. So I started looking for courses at the Fashion Institute of Technology (FIT), where I taught. They had a series of courses in hat-making.

The first class I had to take was blocking—you learn to mold a felt hat onto wooden blocks. I started seeing that hats could be very nice for hair that is starting to grow back in a different texture. Also, my own hair was slow-growing. Making these hats, I realized that short hair actually carries hats very well. I started loving hats myself.

In that class, we didn't learn how to make fabric hats, which I had originally wanted to. I had to take other courses to learn to make a turban-type fabric hat. Now I have a pretty good design. I give samples to friends with cancer and hair loss, requesting they give me feedback. What do they think about the hats? Eventually, hopefully, I can bring these to production.

I also have a prototype for clothing that I created with a student. At FIT, many students are young and female. I was diagnosed with cancer very young, and I learned that young cancer patients have unique challenges. They are in the middle of building their career and family, trying to decide what to do in the future. Then, cancer hits. It's very shocking. I wanted my students to be aware that cancer doesn't affect only the elderly. I wanted to open their eyes to the needs of young cancer patients and to the broader possibilities of fashion inclusiveness.

Fashion isn't only for healthy, young people, I told my class, but for people with cancer, disabilities, and other physical challenges. Fashion can reach out to those populations. To get my students thinking, I showed them my pictures during chemotherapy and said, "This is what I did to let fashion help cancer patients." One of the students responded that she was looking for a project to work on for her senior thesis. She suggested that we could make garments to help breast cancer patients. I was very excited by the idea, and we started working on different types of garments for women recovering from mastectomies, to help them get dressed independently. The garment we created looks very professional and fashionable, but it's comfortable and easy to put on. You can look nice to go to the doctor's office or have lunch with friends. I want cancer patients to be able to go out and feel good about themselves in these garments. So that's my project now.

The Artist's Metamorphosis

· ·

Name: Lelah

Location: Hudson Valley, New York

Diagnosis: Hodgkin's lymphoma; breast cancer

Age at diagnosis: 31, then 41

Age now: 45

I was two years out of grad school, and I had started working with my very first art gallery. I liked storytelling, exploring the fantastical and the dark. I was flourishing in my work and grateful to be making an income doing it. I was living in NYC. I shared an art studio with some friends. I was in a relationship. We had our issues, but that was something I held in and didn't talk about with anyone. Since I held things in, close to my chest, I may always wonder if that contributed to my first round of illness.

BEST ADVICE: The only way to get past it is to go right through it.

At first you want to understand what the cause could be. Was there mold in my studio? Was it genetic? I did past-life-regression therapy to see if it was connected to something beyond my lifetime. I was a little bit reckless with the way I was painting. I was using oil paint, and it would get on my skin.

My boyfriend and I parted ways. Just a few months after, I was diagnosed with Hodgkin's lymphoma, stage 3, and was prescribed ABVD chemo and possibly radiation. In the end, after much deliberation and consulting, I opted not to do the radiation. Oddly, all my tumors were in my chest. It was a very strange coincidence, because ever since I was an infant, I've been sensitive about anyone or anything touching my chest. It's a specific four-inch area, dead center from the throat chakra to the heart chakra—and that's exactly where all my tumors were. I felt as if something mysterious, long with me in looming spirit, had finally arrived in actuality.

Despite having symptoms of late-stage cancer, I didn't realize something was off until I found a weird bump near my collarbone. I immediately walked to the hospital from the movie theater I was in when I discovered it. They took an x-ray and told me "It's nothing," but I insisted until I found a doctor who figured it out. That doctor said, "We're sending you to the ENT right now. We think this is serious." It turned out that I had seven tumors the size of tangerines in my chest.

It took a few weeks before we knew what kind of cancer it was. I either had lymphoma or lung cancer, and I knew lung cancer was going to be more dire. Those two weeks of waiting were difficult. Once we discovered it was lymphoma, it was a relief. I thought, *OK. I can handle this.* But I was dealing with a lot of advanced-stage symptoms: night sweats, fever every afternoon, severe exhaustion, weight loss.

My mother had come up from Florida to live with me in New York. To my friends I was open about what was happening, and people came out of the woodwork to support me, although not everyone knew how. Thankfully, I received money through art grants. And very quickly I was ushered into the most deeply strange phase of my life. The ABVD chemo combination was horrendous and aggressive. I tasted metal, felt dizzy all the time. We cut the "V," Velban, after I experienced respiratory issues. My oncologist did this after my insistence and research, even though all my respiratory tests said there was nothing abnormal.

The tumors were gone three months into chemo, but we had to finish the protocol. Funny, I remember the day I got that news—and how it felt weird, because I wasn't sure what it meant that one day things could seem normal again.

During treatment I was often incapacitated, depending on what phase of chemo I was in. Sometimes I didn't have the energy to walk across the room, and I slept most of the time. I went out occasionally, but that was only right before the next chemo. I saw others and wondered at how well they seemed to function during treatment. The drugs gave me rosy cheeks. Somehow I was well suited to having no hair, and I never covered up my head. I even kept my head shaved for some time after. But meanwhile, I was dealing with hemorrhoids, vomiting, and colossal nausea. I was shitting blood for months and crying on the toilet from discomfort, just to name a few of the unpleasant side effects. You have the chemo drugs, and then you have a tier of drugs to help combat the side effects of those drugs, and then you have maybe alternative meds to help with those side effects. So, you're constantly treating another side effect and taking on another side effect—and then trying to eat well, but often unable to eat at all. I had a shameless hunger for Big Macs and mac and cheese.

The best metaphor to describe the physiological experience is being an insect. Chemo made me think and feel like I was made of iridescent shell and green blood, rather than skin and flesh—that my arteries throughout my system were visible, that I could be easily crushed like a fly. I wasn't a woman. I wasn't human. This was my existence. I tasted metal, I felt small, recovery seemed leagues away, and I was shit-scared. Broken down to something I couldn't form words for and was too tired to express. Bored sometimes, I discovered that Ambien acts similarly to the drug Ecstasy—if you stayed up and didn't lay down. I would occasionally make visitors take it with me.

As treatment finished, I entered a new phase: instability and fear of the outdoors. I didn't ride the subway for months, and the thought of it terrified me beyond anything else. I was lucky. I had a great support system, and I was in a safe, loving environment that I didn't like to leave. Despite the isolation, I felt oddly cozy at home, where I could disappear. People would cook for me. I had my mother there. I just went inside of myself, and the door was shut, until later. There was much safety in that.

The really tough part started with the aftermath—picking up the shell, preparing to reintegrate.

In a perfect world, if I could redo it, I would have hibernated for at least another six months after treatment. I should not have traveled. I should not have done some of the things I did, because my system was not ready for it. I learned the hard way. There will be consequences from jumping too quickly with an immune system that's compromised.

Many people say that post chemo, they felt like a shell of a person. I looked sick and tattered. After treatment, I spent some time in Florida with my parents. While there, I walked into an ashram and I met a master who became a lifelong friend and teacher. I got into kundalini at that time. This master helped me to meditate and heal, and I went into that very deeply. These practices and this master were and still are very important parts of my life.

Every year that passed, I thought—I'm better. But after two or three years, I realized, "Holy shit. This really fucked me up." I think it takes at minimum two to three years to come back physically. It took me a lot longer to recover emotionally—and in a way, I'm not sure how I did. You're always managing that fear of a recurrence.

Last week, I heard about an acquaintance who had cancer at the same time as I did. We both recovered—and then suddenly she had a recurrence, and it took her life. Things like that put you on eggshells, with nightmares and insomnia. Other things that do that to me are excessive alcohol consumption and bad eating habits, logical or not. Nothing is more scary than the shit coming back.

Cancer is a trauma. I didn't realize that until later. What I went through was the most traumatizing thing I ever experienced. It took a long time not to see myself as that sick girl, damaged goods. For a long time it really affected how I thought of myself and how I thought others saw me. I was like, "Who would want to be close to me? I'm not someone who's probably going to last." It was very hard for me just to live and see myself as a viable person, capable of living as long as the next.

I started making art again immediately after chemo. It started with a film in my bedroom. It was shot in time lapse and hooked up to computers, so I could lay in bed while it happened. It was an animation—an erotic film featuring orange peels I cut into human forms and allowed to dry, in a miniature domestic dwelling I made. I was obsessed with death and mortality—and also eroticism, since I had very little libido from the chemo.

I went to Austria for an artist's residency for a few years. It was great. When I returned from Europe, I realized that living in the city was no longer for me.

Funny as this may sound, I decided that my dedication to the art I had been making was ruining my life. So I got rid of my studio and left NYC forever. I moved to the countryside and began to sew and make clothing. Sewing was a sacred, calming hobby I'd had since childhood. I was having an existential crisis of sorts. My art just felt too personal, a very emotional process that I took way too seriously; and it was threatening my happiness. I didn't feel like going to a studio, gutting myself every day, putting it back inside, and then coming home.

I soon started a company of all hand-painted clothing, and it took off. I bought a house. I was in the works to have a child on my own. I made a plan with a midwife and started to prepare. At a visit, she noticed a pea-size bump under my arm. She took a look and said, "I think you should get that checked out."

Of course, I checked it out. There was not one iota of thought in my mind that it could be cancer. It just couldn't. No way. And sure enough, it was cancer. I had breast cancer—stage 1 lobular carcinoma. Not lymphoma; this was not a recurrence.

I did not have an aggressive cancer, but it was hormone sensitive. I was prescribed radiation and tamoxifen—undoubtedly, a huge impediment for my fertility.

Since I had been around this block already, although with a different cancer, I wasn't prepared to experience all the feelings I'd had before.

My first lumpectomy was botched. The morning of the surgery, I'd opened my closet door—the bottom of the broom fell forward and scraped my eye, scratching my cornea. This burned like bloody hell. There wasn't time to deal with it; I had to go straight to the breast surgery. I had local anesthesia, and we soon discovered my immunity to Lidocaine. I was awake and crying throughout the entire surgery, asking for more shots of local anesthesia, because I could feel the procedure taking place.

It turned out the surgeon had not gotten clear margins. And the way she gave me the news that I had cancer was less than ideal. I remember going into a rage at the hospital, screaming as I felt the dreadful envelope of shock that only bad, bad news can bring. After that news, like a zombie, I had to go straight to the eye clinic.

I ended up going to Sloan Kettering for a second surgery to clear the margins. I saw numerous oncologists and radiologists and surgeons. I wanted someone to tell me I didn't have to go through this nightmare again. It didn't happen that way, but I was insistent. I tried going holistic for a whole year after the lumpectomy. I was in a hospital in Germany. I went on radical diets and changed my lifestyle—and thus discovered I wasn't able to sustain the hardcore path that demanded. So I changed course and went with the original prescribed course of action, only a year later. I realized that to go holistic and treat cancer, you've got to be militant. I felt I was too young to be that strict, and it didn't fit who I was.

I ended up doing radiation and going on the tamoxifen. Most radiologists and oncologists thought it was too late for me to do radiation. I saw some of the best doctors, and some gasped at the fact that I'd tried an alternative route and didn't want any part of my future treatment. Finally I found a radiologist I loved and an oncologist I felt good about.

After a year of tamoxifen, I told my oncologist I still wanted to have a child and that I had frozen eggs. She said, "You know, I know how much that would help you, so I'm going to let you get off tamoxifen because I don't think you're in danger. I'm not worried, but you have 18 months to get off and do something about it, and then you're getting right back on the tamoxifen."

Despite my efforts and desires, having a child in my own body didn't work out. It was the biggest, hardest, most jagged pill I ever had to swallow, something I once felt shame and a lot of grief over.

Prior to breast cancer, I had strong self-esteem and confidence. Afterward, not only did I lose it, but it went into the negative. I went through shame and the difficult sense that my illness would outweigh my presence. It was prominent in my psyche, and there were times when I felt like an utter failure in every respect. It led to serious depression over the years and suicidal periods. But over time I graduated into a much different place, becoming another kind of strong. Acceptance had a lot to do with that. Before, I would not have willingly put this all out there—but I know the strength it may give someone else to hear this vulnerability and another person's story. Undoubtedly, there's a strength in vulnerability.

I made the decision to adopt rather than conceive on my own. I started to get really scared about recurrence, since my cancer was hormone-sensitive. Cancer is fucking smart and has a mind of its own.

My path meandered back to making art and fully enjoying it again. That's my lifeline. It's always been my lifeline. I tried to lose it for a while, but that was impossible. You just can't alter who you are.

I had to come up with a very different relationship to my work. I finally had the realization that, OK, I can actually make art without entirely losing myself emotionally in it. But I had to work with who I was and what I needed to be—and I'm not exactly that same person I used to be, and naturally some things have changed in the way I work. That's also what an artist must do: Invent; reinvent. Taking five years away from my life's work was essential to my reinterpretation and restaging.

Progress with making art has helped me feel stronger over the years. One tiny little success leads to another little something. To turn the tables sometimes, just don't dwell too long, and keep going.

Reimagining the Pink Ribbon

Name: Dorkys Ramos

Town: New York, New York

Diagnosis: Breast cancer

Age at diagnosis: 30, then 34

Age Now: 37

When I was first diagnosed with breast cancer, in December 2012, I was so reluctant to let cancer change anything in my life. Instead of having my lumpectomy right away, I scheduled the surgery for the first week of January, because I still wanted to enjoy my holidays. I had also launched my own stationery company, Porcupine Hugs, just two weeks before my diagnosis, and all I wanted to do in those days was grow my greeting-card collection. I was glad I'd created my company before I was diagnosed, because I didn't want anyone to say cancer was a catalyst for positive changes in my life or that it motivated this creative pursuit. I didn't want cancer to get any of the credit.

My diagnosis came completely out of left field, because I was so young and I don't have a family history of breast cancer. But I just kept on and filled my days with drawing, working, and freelance writing. When I had my lumpectomy, I took the weekend off and then went right back to work on Monday. I was still bandaged up and typing stories one-handed on my laptop, but I just did not want to stop. Looking back, it probably wasn't the healthiest move, but returning to my "normal life" is what I needed in order to cope with my scary reality.

BEST ADVICE: If I could, I would tell my pre-diagnosis self not to be afraid of letting cancer change me. The first time around, I really dug my heels into the ground and refused to do anything differently, even if it would be for my own good. But after the second diagnosis, I was more open to making positive changes. This time, I'm doing a better job of taking care of me.

After my lumpectomy, I got the results of my genetic testing and learned the cancer wasn't gene-based—which was good, because otherwise my treatment would have been much harsher. In February 2016, I started radiation, and the exhaustion finally caught up with me. Radiation drained my energy, and I was so sleepy all the time. I was angry that I couldn't stay up as late as I needed to finish something; and commuting to the cancer center every day for three weeks straight really wore on me. It was a low point, with a lot of feeling sorry for myself—and blaming myself, as if it were my fault I was exhausted.

And still, I found myself plowing through life. I really dove into my art. That holiday season, I had released the first three cards from my company. By April, I had more than 20 cards. Painting with watercolors and creating art became my therapy, and it was all you'd find me doing, every free moment I had. My illustrations are very whimsical and serve as my escape. The cute little scenes I create help bring some color into this darkness.

Later on that year, I created a breast cancer card with my own version of the pink ribbon, because I didn't feel like that ribbon truly symbolized my experience. The pink ribbon looks so pretty and perfect, and here I was feeling like crap. So I created a ribbon that starts out pink and pretty—but by the time it reaches the other end, it's tattered and brown. It was my way of visualizing the two ends of this illness. There are some positives that come with being in this situation, one being that you can better relate to and feel deep empathy for others who are going through something similar. Sometimes things seem very hopeful, and you're getting all this support from family and friends. But then at other times, you're in this dark hole, and it sucks, and you don't want people to tell you it's going to be OK, because you know what? You don't know. You don't know if it's going to be OK. No one can promise that.

Even when the cancer was treated, I was always certain that it would come back. There was no piece of me that thought that it was "a one and done," because I was still so young. It's not like I was diagnosed at 70. I had a lot of time for things to go wrong again, so that was always in the back of my mind. I just didn't know it would come back so soon.

In September of 2016, four years after my initial diagnosis, I went in for my regular appointment, and my oncology surgeon felt a lump under my left armpit. She immediately sent me upstairs to have a quick biopsy. Before I knew it, I was laying back on the table and having a needle injected into the lump. When I cried out, it wasn't just from the pain; I was terrified of what might come next. The doctor performing the biopsy asked me, "Are you crying because it hurts or because you're upset?"

"It's everything!" I sobbed. "I'm crying over everything."

When I saw the surgeon again a few minutes later, she confirmed that my worst fear had come true: I had breast cancer again.

Within a week, I was having another lumpectomy. Since the cancer I had feeds on estrogen to grow, I began hormonal therapy, to decrease the amount of estrogen my body produces. To this day, I take Lupron injections every month, in addition to the daily tamoxifen pills I've been taking since 2013. In the beginning it was awful, because of the constant hot flashes— Lupron forces your body into chemical menopause. Thankfully, the side effects have eased up over time.

Unfortunately, the pathology results from my surgery brought bad news: The margins were not clear from the lumpectomy, which meant I'd need another one in order to have a high probability that all cancer cells were removed from the area. Then one of my doctors called me and said, "Listen, we think that you should consider a mastectomy."

Again, I completely lost it. I wasn't ready to accept that such a drastic measure would be necessary to keep me alive and that from then on my body would look different. It's been two and a half years, and I'm still learning to accept my new body.

I opted for a double mastectomy, because God forbid I'd have to go through this process again if I developed cancer in my other breast. I scheduled the surgery for the beginning of December 2016. The weeks leading up to that day were tough to say the least—so much crying and sobbing. The morning of the procedure, I was crying in bed, crying in the shower, crying on our way to the hospital. I couldn't believe I was going to go through with it. Knowing this was the right choice for me didn't make it any easier to do. I'm so glad I had been going to therapy for my anxiety and depression, because it also helped me cope with this second round of cancer.

When I said goodbye to my family and my boyfriend before the nurse walked me to the operating room, I was simultaneously trembling and sobbing and trying so hard to be brave. The incredible thing was that after all that crying I did on my walk to the operating room, I don't remember crying at all once I woke up from the surgery—not in the hospital, anyway. It felt like a testament to how resilient the human mind can be. It's like a switch turned on, and my brain said, "OK, this is our reality now." Physically, it was painful. I felt like I'd been run over by an 18-wheeler, or as if my top half were encased in cement. I couldn't shift my position in bed or pee without someone's help. I couldn't lift certain things, reach overhead, open heavy doors, or even put on a coat, because I couldn't bend my arms back. I couldn't do anything for myself, and I had to relinquish a lot of control. It was very frustrating for someone who struggles with asking for help.

I chose to have immediate breast reconstruction. During the same surgery as the mastectomy, a plastic surgeon inserted expanders into my chest, and over the course of the year, these "balloons" were gradually filled to make room for the more permanent breast implants. I was slated for five weeks of radiation and a regimen of tamoxifen pills and Lupron injections that continues to this day.

As much as it pained me, I had to back out of holiday markets that year. I always help organize an annual event with this group of Etsy sellers from the tristate area, but with the mastectomy in the beginning of December, I just couldn't do it. Still, I refused to stay put; so the Friday after my mastectomy, I went to the crowded event, just to say hello to people and cheer them on. I was so scared of people bumping into me—but I didn't want to be home all the time, and I wanted to give the impression of "See? I am totally OK. This was nothing," even though the reality was completely different.

With my first diagnosis at 30 years old, I was told I wouldn't be able to get pregnant during my five years of treatment. Even though I'd been torn about having kids, losing that choice was a really hard pill to swallow. Eventually, I thought, *OK, I can take these next five years and do all the things that I want for myself, become more financially stable, and feel more fulfilled. Then, in five years, I'll be better prepared to raise a child.* But four years later, cancer happened again—and at that point, I had to pull my head out of the sand and actively confront my fears and options regarding my fertility. Five more years of treatment would mean I'd be trying to conceive at nearly 40 years old.

So last summer, I decided to freeze my eggs. I'm scared of needles and never thought I'd willingly inject myself every night just to have a child someday. But I did it—to have some control over this part of my life. It's not 100% guaranteed I'll be able to have kids, but this was better than doing nothing at all. I keep referring to "future Dorkys" when I do things I don't really want to do at the moment, knowing that Dorkys in the future will appreciate the pain I'm going through now.

Saying the last six years have been a freaking roller-coaster would be an understatement. My bucket is always filled to the brim, and if any little thing goes wrong, I overflow and start crying. I'm working on accepting that there's a legitimate physical, mental, and emotional toll this has taken on me, even if it's not visible from the outside. Through it all, art and writing have been my salvation. When I paint, I escape into my own little happy zone. Nothing bad can happen to me there.

Ultimate Frisbee for the Win

· ·

Name: Elana Schwam

Town: Cambridge, Massachusetts

Diagnosis: Malignant melanoma; stage 3

Age at diagnosis: 29

Age now: 32

I was diagnosed with stage 3B metastatic melanoma on June 28th, 2016. If you Google metastatic melanoma, it assumes you have stage 4 and gives you something like a 10% chance of survival, so this couldn't have been more terrifying. The diagnosis came as a total shock. I was probably in my best shape ever at the time, working out and feeling great. Plus I didn't have any suspicious moles—which is where melanoma comes from. My life revolved around my intensive graduate-level nursing program, my boyfriend, and my Ultimate Frisbee team, Brute Squad.

Brute Squad is not your average Ultimate team. We are playing at the highest level possible: We're a nationally ranked team representing the city of Boston. I had been playing with Brute Squad for four years. Before cancer, I'd been drawn to Ultimate for two reasons. One, it was the most fun sport I had ever played. I didn't pick up Ultimate until halfway through college; before that, I was a basketball player and a college soccer goalie. I was always more skilled with my hands than with my feet. I loved running, chasing after the disc—and I was a natural at laying out (when you dive to catch or block the disc), so it was the perfect thing for me. And two, the Ultimate Frisbee community is the most welcoming, supportive environment I have ever experienced. Ultimate accepts every kind of person, and the women Ultimate players embraced each other and celebrated each other as badass athletes. I had been on a lot of sports teams throughout my life, but every Ultimate team I've been on has been special, especially Brute Squad. The team made up my closest friends, and I looked forward to practice every weekend. We were all intelligent, strong, motivated, silly, and united at striving toward a common goal: to win another national championship.

> BEST ADVICE: Everyone needs something different, but my advice would be to continue to live your life as you normally would. Surround yourself with people and things that you love, and live it up. Obviously, there are days where you need to cry and just watch Netflix on the couch all day. But I found that the busier I stayed and the more I filled my life, the better I felt and functioned.

My cancer story actually started six years prior to my diagnosis. I discovered a new itchy, irregular mole on my back when I was a senior in college, back in 2010. I went to a dermatologist when I was home for Christmas break who thought it was irregular enough to biopsy. The biopsy came back as a spitz nevus, which is a type of benign (noncancerous) mole. My dermatologist said something like, "Sometimes these things are confused with cancer, so we take out the mole with extra skin just to be safe."

I didn't think anything of it at the time. I was busy with writing my capstone thesis and captaining my college Ultimate team. They removed the mole, and I went back to my life. I never thought about it unless people asked me about the scar. Fast forward to the spring of 2016. I was writing a paper for school about the epidemiology of breast cancer, and I decided to perform a breast exam on myself. To my surprise, I found a pea-size lump just under my armpit. When you're in school related to a health profession, there's a phenomenon of wanting to diagnose yourself with everything you read about. I tried to stay cool, but in the back of my mind I was terrified. I brought it up to my PCP during my yearly physical, and she said, "It's probably nothing, but I'll refer you to a surgeon just in case." The surgeon said, "It's probably nothing, but if you want, we can do an ultrasound." The ultrasound tech was concerned during the exam and went and got the radiologist—who came in for five seconds and said, "What we are worried about in this clinic is cancer, and what you have is just a cyst."

Over three months' time, my little lump had grown from a pea to a marble, clearly visible when I raised my arm. I had a bad feeling in the pit of my stomach, so I decided to have it removed anyway for peace of mind. When the doctor called me to her office after the surgery, I thought it was just protocol. Instead she said, "We had a surprise. It turns out that it was in fact a lymph node that was essentially taken over by a tumor, and it's testing positive for melanoma."

I couldn't believe that everyone had told me it was nothing and that I actually had the worst-case scenario, which was cancer. I was a wreck in the room, sobbing. I got even worse when my father, who's an emergency-room physician and usually a "cool as a cucumber" type, cursed out loud when the doctor read him the pathology report. The rest of the day I spent getting a CT scan of my abdomen, chest, and pelvis. They didn't warn me that you get this intense burning sensation when they inject the dye, so I wrongly thought it was an indication that the cancer was everywhere.

That was Tuesday. Wednesday was spent making appointments with oncologists, and communicating with the dermatologist who had removed the spitz nevus from my back six years earlier, in hopes that the new melanoma diagnosis was wrong. I found out a week later that it was actually the dermatologist who had misdiagnosed me. It had been melanoma six years before. They had removed it all, but the shitty thing about melanoma is that it can lie dormant for years and then recur.

By Thursday, I was exhausted from thinking about cancer. All I wanted was to decompress in my apartment with my boyfriend and think about something other than cancer. My boyfriend and I had a summer-league Ultimate Frisbee game that night, but I also had a brain MRI scheduled at 10 p.m. The game was actually on the way to the MRI clinic, so I said, "Let's just go and play while I still can." I realized something while I was out there running around: This was the first time my brain had stopped thinking about cancer. A lightbulb went on in my head: This is what would get me through my months and months of treatment. Ultimate was the one thing I could do to completely clear my mind. Going that night, in the middle of my diagnosis, was the best thing I could have done. I realized then that I wanted to keep playing as long as I could, whatever happened with my treatment.

That weekend, Brute Squad had a three-day tournament in Rhode Island. I emailed the Brute Squad leadership and the rest of the team and told them of my diagnosis. I didn't know what my status for the season would be, I added, but I was going to play my heart out in the tournament with them that coming weekend.

After meeting with the oncologist the Monday after, I found out that the first part of my treatment would be surgery to remove more tissue under my arm. When I had the lump removed, before we knew it was cancer, she had taken the tumor out in pieces—not something you want to do with a tumor. They also planned a wider excision on my back, where the original melanoma had been. I was super worried that I was going to miss playing in a big tournament in Colorado a week and a half later. Before the surgery, I spoke with the surgeon about wanting to be able to play in the tournament. He said he could use an older type of stitches that were stronger and left more of a scar but would allow me to get back on the field quicker. I didn't think twice about that. I had never missed a tournament, and the thought of not being able to be with my teammates, playing the sport I loved, was devastating—especially now that it was my main source of therapy. I was going to do everything I could to make sure I was on that plane to Colorado. So I did the older stitches and played the tournament, and it was awesome. I wanted to play as much as possible before I started a drug protocol for melanoma a month later.

For treatment, I ended up going with the cancer center at Massachusetts General Hospital (MGH). My treatment team was amazing. I loved them. Chemotherapy doesn't have an effect on melanoma. There has been a lot of new, exciting research surrounding immunotherapy, and there were a lot of clinical trials I could consider. Jimmy Carter had stage 4 melanoma and went on one of these trial drugs, called Keytruda—and he now has no evidence of disease. In the years before these immunotherapies, stage 4 melanoma was pretty much a death sentence.

So I entered a clinical trial, hoping to get this miracle drug. But instead I was randomized to the standard treatment, which is interferon. Interferon is terrible. It's an old treatment for hepatitis C. I had infusions five days a week for a month. My treatment was a little different because my liver was not tolerating it well, so I kept having to take breaks. After the main bulk of the treatment, you're supposed to give yourself subcutaneous injections three times a week for the rest of the year.

Interferon makes you feel like you have the flu. It gives you high fevers, body aches, depression, fatigue, everything. It's a shitty treatment. It's exhausting. Technology and science with immunotherapies and melanoma is changing so fast. They don't use interferon anymore at all, really—because it doesn't have much of a benefit and the side effects, while they are self-limiting, pretty much put you out for a year.

Yet somehow, I was able to play the entire Ultimate season while on interferon. The first few days each week were the worst, if I didn't take Tylenol around the clock. If I slept through a dose, I was dealing with the worst flu symptoms you could imagine: body aches, rigors, nausea, vomiting, pounding headache. But if I stayed on top of my Tylenol regimen, later in the week all I felt was a little fatigue. They were giving me tons of fluid via IV. Before interferon, I must have been chronically dehydrated, because after the IV hydration I felt like superwoman. I was crushing it at practice, and everyone was like, "What the hell? Why is Schwam getting better at Ultimate during cancer treatment?"

As the month went on, however, interferon started to take its toll on me. At Nationals, I was a shell of myself as an athlete, which was really hard because I had been working my ass off that season. I was barely able to keep up when I was on the field. Usually I was known for my tight, aggressive defense and my ability to run nonstop. But at Nationals I was just trying to survive, and it was miserable. I was terrified of letting my team down but also wanted to be out there and contribute. Before every tournament, my oncologist would say, "This is probably the last tournament you can play in" because of fatigue. But I kept proving him wrong. I'd had ongoing discussions with the captains and coach throughout the season, and I never once asked them to limit my playing time—quite the opposite. But at Nationals, for the first time, they could see that I was struggling. My playing time decreased, and that was OK. I wanted our team to perform the best that we could, even though sitting out was personally devastating. In the end we won our back-to-back National Championship—and in our final team picture, my team wore these custom tanks they had made to support me. It was a surprise, and it was incredible to have so much support. Players from other teams were also reaching out to me right and left, sending me good wishes and words of encouragement. I was nominated for an award, and even ESPN announcers reached out to me, to feature my story during the game.

After Nationals, I completely fell apart. It was a mixture of the Ultimate season ending and the cumulative effects of the interferon catching up with me. I was exhausted and deeply depressed. I didn't see my teammates every weekend as I had during the Ultimate season. I had a long off-season of cancer treatment ahead of me. Just before I was about to shift to the maintenance version of interferon, I went in for an appointment. I was teary with my oncologist, and my parents were so worried about my change in affect. My oncologist had never seen me so down; he knew me as the crazy Ultimate

Frisbee player who would stop at nothing. But there I was, barely doing school work, barely even able to take a shower. It was bad.

Science meanwhile had been moving so quickly that my oncologist came back from a conference and told me, "They just released new data from a new study." They had found that this other immunotherapy called ipilimumab, under the trade name Yervoy, has better long-term results for melanoma—significantly better in terms of disease-free survival and long-term recurrence prevention. He switched me to that treatment. The downside of Yervoy is it has a lot of serious, bad side effects. You have an infusion every three weeks, for four or five total infusions, and then you have one every three months for three years. But something like 80% of patients on the drug don't make it through the first four infusions without some sort of autoimmune reaction, such as colitis.

So I started Yervoy. I was scared because of all the things that can go wrong. I had one infusion; it went well. There were a couple of random days where I had a mild fever, but other than that it was fine compared to interferon. Since the Ultimate season was over, I was just in school. School was hard because it was mentally exhausting and often made me think more about my cancer. I would end up going down research rabbit holes, trying to figure out my chances of recurrence. I had an incredibly supportive boyfriend and family and would see my Ultimate friends—but way less than during the season. At least school was incredibly time-consuming, and staying busy helped.

Unfortunately though, after my second infusion with Yervoy, I had a terrible autoimmune reaction and liver injury that caused raging fevers, rigors, and night sweats for a week until they treated me with prednisone for about two months. So that was the end of Yervoy—and my abrupt end of cancer treatment. I was declared "no evidence of disease" after my first couple of surgeries, but since melanoma at my stage has such a high recurrence rate (50-60% over five years), they typically do preventative immunotherapy. Given my bad reaction, my oncologist decided instead to rely on frequent surveillance imaging. I continue to have full-body CT scans and brain MRIs every four months and still have no evidence of disease. I will likely continue these scans, but over a longer interval, for the next 10 years.

Meanwhile, the science of immunotherapy keeps moving forward. They don't even treat with Yervoy anymore. They have found other immunotherapies that are more effective and safer. It's comforting to know that if I do have a recurrence, science has a few more tricks up its sleeve.

Had I not played Ultimate through most of my treatment, I would have been thinking about cancer all the time. It would have been a much more miserable experience and much harder to move on from. I also continued with my grad program and am grateful that I did. My instinct was that I needed to keep living life. I felt this intensity around it. When Ultimate ended I was so sad, but over time I learned other ways of coping.

Being physically active has always been a huge part of maintaining my mental health. Throughout this process, I had been blogging about my experience, which was also very therapeutic for me. Now that I had no evidence of disease, I realized I not only wanted but needed to do more to prevent this illness from happening to other people. Writing on my blog about prevention was no longer enough. I signed up to run the Boston Marathon for charity, in support of the New England organization IMPACT Melanoma. IMPACT is a nonprofit whose mission is to reduce incidences of melanoma through education about prevention and patient support. I ended up raising almost $14,000. I continue to share my story wherever I can, to spread awareness about the dangers of melanoma and information on preventing it. I spoke at the IMPACT Melanoma Gala this fall and helped raise more money than I can even comprehend. I have been interviewed on Ultimate podcasts and am in the process of writing other pieces.

The other thing that has helped me the most post-treatment is Project Koru. After treatment, I was terrified of recurrence and felt more alone than ever before. It was relatively easy to be actively fighting cancer, but then I felt like I was just waiting for the cancer to come back. I also had a lot of guilt about not being happier that I had no evidence of disease. I realized with the help of therapists that I was traumatized from my experience.

Project Koru is an organization that helps give young-adult cancer survivors meaning in their lives after cancer. It provides week-long surfing or skiing trips free to survivors and helps young-adult survivors connect with one another.

My trip to Camp Koru was an incredible experience. Until then, I didn't know anyone else within decades of my age who'd had cancer. I found out that everyone felt similar to me. They too were having a tough time re-adjusting to normal life. They too were scared every day about recurrence. They too felt guilty for being cancer-free and still being scared. They too had families and friends who didn't understand why they couldn't just be happy with their lives, knowing they currently didn't have cancer. Just knowing I was not alone was more than enough for me to kickstart my life again. I was inspired to become a leader and volunteer at Camp Koru, so I can help provide a similar healing opportunity to other young cancer survivors. The experience has been so incredible and at the same time therapeutic for me as well.

Now I am a primary-care nurse practitioner, providing health care to underserved patients in a community-health setting. Recently I had to inform a patient that they had cancer. Having my own personal experience with illness has definitely made me a better nurse practitioner and motivat-ed me to be more empathetic. I'll also never brush off a seemingly young, healthy patient who says there is something wrong with their body. Oh, also, I married that awesome boyfriend of mine in August 2018, and I continue to play Ultimate for Brute Squad. I feel incredibly lucky and am so grateful for the incredible Ultimate community, my family, and my husband, Aaron.

Hero's Beads

· ·

Name: Katie Smith

Town: Wilmington, Delaware

Diagnosis: Oligodendroglioma (brain tumor); grade two

Age at diagnosis: 32

Age now: 37

On October 7th, 2013, I was awoken at 1 a.m. by my partner, Ann Marie, who was urging me to put on my bra so we could go downstairs and open the door for the ambulance. I started crying—I'm afraid of ambulances—and asked her why. "I think you had a seizure," she said.

Ann Marie had asked me, pleaded with me, so many times in the past to stop playing pranks on her. I'd fake getting struck by lightning. I'd fake getting shocked while unplugging cords. It was certainly in my bag of sick jokes to fake a seizure. But I wasn't faking. I didn't know what a bra was. I couldn't put a bra on. We left the bedroom with me still in my pajamas.

WORST ADVICE: "Don't do radiation or chemo. They are poison." You tell me what you would do when you have a tumor in your brain that is going to get worse and *is* going to kill you if left untreated. I am going to do radiation and chemo. *I* am going to treat my tumor with these chemicals and hope for a cure in the future. In *my* future!

Later, we'd learn she was right: She had watched me have a tonic clonic seizure—what used to be called a grand mal seizure, with full-body convulsions. It was my first but wouldn't be my last. After seizures, I fall into a postictal phase, and I'm confused and disoriented. I couldn't remember the seizure at all that night. I couldn't remember who I was or who *anyone* was. I didn't remember or understand much of anything. Ann Marie still wasn't *quite* sure if I was messing around with her.

Downstairs, Ann Marie handed me my slip-on shoes, but I had no idea what they were or what to do with them. I sat on the stairs in the foyer while she manipulated my limp feet into my shoes like I was a toddler. My emotions were unstable. I cycled through terror, disbelief, confusion, and irritation. When the paramedics arrived, the male EMT asked the normal questions: "What is your name?" *Katie?* "What year is it?" *2012?* The EMT was all business. "No, it's actually 2013. What is your address?" *15…uh…15…I don't know. Ask her!* I pointed at Ann Marie. "No," the EMT said. "I need to hear it from you." *You just drove here! You know it!* I had lived in the house for three years by then, but I couldn't recall the address. *I don't know it.* Next question from the EMT: "Do you know who this young lady is beside you?" This one confused me too. I said, *Yes. But I can't remember her name. I know I love her.* Then he asked me if I knew who our president was. Ah! This was the one question I knew with certainty. With a big grin, I said, *Obama!*

As we walked out the door, I asked the EMT if I was going to die. He said, "Well, we're all going to die sometime, but right now, we're just going to get you checked out to see what's going on." This terrified me, and I cried hard. Inside the ambulance was a new EMT, this one still training. I was crying and repeating, "I'm so scared." I think she might have broken protocol when she asked if I wanted her to hold my hand. I did want that, and holding her hand made me feel so much better.

We went to the smaller of our city's two hospitals, because it had the shortest wait time. I'll always have a special place in my heart for the doctor who calmly and quietly pulled up a chair and delivered the results of my CT scan in a gentle and apologetic voice. "We have the results," she said. "There is a mass in your brain."

That's when the blood rushed to my ears and I couldn't hear anymore. I went to that place that you go when you're told you are going to die—and pretty soon, actually. Not when you're old and feeble and can't walk on your own. No. For you, Katie Smith, age 32, for you, you're going to die very soon. They saw it on the scan—a mass in my brain. Fuck. I was just told by complete strangers that I had a seizure. I still had no idea what the hell *that* was. I wasn't in my body when it *allegedly* convulsed. In fact, I felt like I couldn't be sure that I'd actually had a seizure. It was still dark outside. That meant that there was still a chance that none of this was real—that I was asleep. If this was still happening when tomorrow came, then I'd have to start to believe it was real.

Obviously, it was true. All of it. Well, all of it except the part about dying. That was never said; it's just what my fear told me. At this point, nobody knew what kind of tumor it was.

I decided against having surgery at the local hospital and was taken by a special neuro-ambulance to a leading hospital in Philadelphia. There, I interviewed a highly recommended neurosurgeon. I liked that I got to pick my own surgeon. I think my family was put off by his blunt personality, but I picked this man precisely because he was gruff. I appreciated that he didn't go out of his way to be polite. It felt like this qualified him to take on my tumor.

And so, there I was, my forehead autographed by my surgeon, having conversations with each of my family members. It wasn't said, but those talks were crucial to my family and me in the event that I didn't make it. Ann Marie walked in pace with my gurney back to surgery, never once letting go of my hand. She is everything to me. She reassured me repeatedly that everything was going to be fine. I said, "Yeah, but how will I find you in heaven if it's not fine? I want to have a plan in place. Nobody ever thinks about it before they die, but I can." Once again, Ann Marie eased my worries when she said,

"Look at me." I did. She continued, "You are not going to die. I am right here by your side, and I'm going to be right here when you wake up."

Ann Marie has a unique way of calming me with her tone when things are too much for me. She stills my panic. On that day and many days ahead, she made the situation seem completely normal. Can you imagine that someone could make brain surgery seem like just another day? Ann Marie rubbed my hand over and over, and it acted as a lullaby. I got my shot of Ativan and started my countdown from 100 to 1, but I actually fell asleep at 99.

I woke up seven hours later from my six-hour-long surgery to see Ann Marie beside me, already holding my hand. I was surprised that I was still alive. My head was wrapped in thick layers of gauze. My total hospital stay, between the two hospitals, was around seven days.

I've heard that when new parents bring their first baby home, they feel like, "Umm...guys...I don't think I should be going home. I have no idea how to do this. What about the nurses and the beeping monitors? Surely they're coming too, right?" This is how I felt when I got home. I was groggy and disoriented. Splitting headaches were my constant companion. Ann Marie was religious about swapping out my ice packs, bringing me my meds, and praying with me, even though neither one of us is religious. We were both scared at night; it took months until we could sleep upstairs in our bedroom, the scene of the event. We slept in the living room, me on a borrowed single bed and Ann Marie on the couch. We would watch Eighties shows, letting Alex P. Keaton and Mr. Belvedere lull us into sleep.

Every day, our house was full of visitors. One of my favorite visits was from my godmother, Elaine, and her grandson, my "nephew," Aiden. Aiden was just nine years old at the time, and he was a survivor of a pediatric brain tumor. He'd been through the whole deal—surgery, radiation, and chemo—when he was just a toddler. Before my surgery, Aiden had visited the hospital and brought me a framed photograph of himself and me from the time I helped him find a four-leaf clover. He'd even pressed his lucky clover between the glass and the photo mat.

Aiden had been through so much. To mark his victories, he had a very long strand of beads. Every bead represented a procedure he had endured. For each procedure—whether he made it through with tears or screams, with restraint, in quarantine, with a port, with a mask, whatever the circumstance—he had a bead to show for it, a bead to remind him that he was courageous. And he was. With his beads as his trophy, Aiden could remember that he was a true hero.

When he visited me at home after surgery, Aiden arrived with a strand of beads that he had selected to represent my own medical triumphs. There was one for my surgery, one for each day in the hospital, one for each of my 30 stitches. At the bottom of the picture he had given me in the hospital, Aiden used cheerfully colored crayons to write, "If I can do it, you can do it!" And so, with my beads, my lucky clover, and inspiration from a child warrior,

I did it.

From December 2013 to July 2015, the entirety of my life was focused on my treatment. When I was first gifted with my beads, the strand was two feet long. By July 2015, it had grown to 19 feet. Like Aiden's, each of my beads represented a specific health or medical experience: surgery, radiation, chemotherapy, ambulance rides, ER visits, doctor visits, blood labs, blood transfusions, MRIs, CTs, IVs, X-rays, fertility treatments, hair loss, hair growth, port placement, port flush, port removal, etc.

When I was home and feeling well enough, I made the beads myself from clay. Making my beads was one thing I could control, and I needed this. When I was making beads, nobody was making decisions for me, tightening my arm with their rubber tourniquet, waking me from my sleep to stab my belly with their needles and leaving bruises, scrubbing my bald head with grit and sticking on electrodes. It was satisfying to look down at my hands and see decisions I had made! Red clay caked in the "life line" in my palm. Pink in my relationship line. Orange in my heart line. Blue clay under my index-finger nail. Yellow in the wrinkle of my middle finger. Green at the bottom of my inner palm. Purple lingering on my chin where I had an itch. All of my beads were unique. The beads brought color into my life, and color is so important to me. I feel that colors manifest health, power, and all things good.

My tumor was a big one at 6 cm, between the size of a golf ball and a tennis ball. Through surgery, my gruff surgeon was able to resect 60-70% of the tumor. Resecting more would have resulted in paralysis of my left side. I like to keep things light and say that the remaining tumor is "in jail" and "on good behavior." I had radiation to create scar tissue to encapsulate what remains and discourage future growth. It has been five years now. In these five years, I've had a total of six seizures. It takes time to find the cocktail of medications for your specific body to keep the seizures at bay. It's still hard. The tumor is in the right frontal lobe, which is responsible for a lot of things, including personality, motivation, emotion regulation, and different types of memory. You might not realize it, but there are lots of types of memory that your brain relies on to get through a day. Some areas of memory and processing that have been affected for me include short-term, long-term, overall processing, executive functioning, and working memory. Basically, I can still do lots of the things I could do before, but I'm very slow, and it's harder to remember new information. The one thing that helps and makes me feel calm is the fact that I can take pictures. They aid me in my keeping my memories close.

When I was in Maui, at Camp Koru, I wandered around the hostel where I stayed prior to the start of camp, capturing loads of pictures. I had never been at a hostel, so I wanted to remember it. In the back there was some kind of an outdoor taco eatery. It was closed, so I had to use my imagination to see the place filled with people, music, tacos, drinks, and the occasional rooster strolling by. Lights were strung; there were pieces of furniture painted ketchup red and mustard yellow. Here and there were fallen leaves and freshly planted flowers swaying in the breeze.

I took a picture of a little pink flower. I debated whether to take the picture—it was just this tiny little thing—but I took it. When I got home I found out that the little flower was a Vinca flower. One of the chemicals used in my chemo was derived from the Vinca plant. I always knew that part of my chemo came from a flower, but I had never actually seen a Vinca flower that I could remember. I had PCV chemo, which stands for Procarbazine, CCNU, and Vincristine. Throughout my journey, I've tried to think of my chemo as helpful, and my radiation, too. I think of them in a positive light. The Vincristine was the worst of the three, in that it made my body very sick. There were days when I couldn't stand up straight because my stomach hurt too much. On those days, I had to walk slumped forward. Knowing that my treatment was made out of a beautiful flower was very helpful to me. And in Hawaii, that flower found me, and I took its picture.

Purpose & Gratitude After Thyroid Cancer

· ·

Name: Vanessa Steil

Location: Long Island, New York

Diagnosis: Papillary thyroid carcinoma

Age at diagnosis: 26

Age now: 32

"*I'm sorry, but you have papillary thyroid carcinoma,*" said the endocrinologist in a monotone voice. If I thought the words seemed to linger on his lips longer than they should have, they took even more time to register in my head. I sat silently and thought, *Well, at least it's not thyroid cancer.*

But that's exactly what it was.

My remaining time with the endocrinologist was a blur. I vaguely remember small fragments of what he said, but I can recall verbatim the "what-ifs" that flashed in my mind. The only edict from the doctor that I clearly recollect were his parting words, a stern warning not to make this diagnosis into a research project. With a sliver of a smile and a final handshake, we parted and I was off on this new journey as a thyroid cancer patient.

Weeks earlier, I had been a healthy, care-free 26-year-old whose only major challenge was mapping out a career plan post-college. The furthest thing from my mind was a cancer diagnosis—let alone hearing that I had cancer in a part of my body whose function I didn't even understand. The words "endocrinologist" and "papillary thyroid carcinoma" were lost on me. I could hardly even comprehend how we'd arrived at this diagnosis. It came about in the most unexpected way.

BEST ADVICE: If I could go back in time and visit that scared 26-year-old girl who thought her life was over, I would tell her that it's just beginning. Even though she wouldn't believe it, I would whisper, "You're going to get through this, and you're going to be a much stronger person for it." And when she does get through it, she will finally understand her presence and her purpose. Her mantra will become: You're stronger than anything in this world that could impede your path.

Prior to my consult with the endocrinologist, I had gone to a gynecologist for what I expected to be a routine exam. It was the first time I'd seen this gynecologist, and after a brief review of my health history, he asked if he could perform a neck check. The question caught me off guard, but I agreed. He checked my neck and said, "Has anyone told you that you have a nodule on the right side of your thyroid?" I shook my head, and he tried to allay my fears by saying it was likely benign. Still, he said, I should have blood drawn and go for a neck ultrasound to confirm that was the case. His response put my mind at ease, for the time being.

A month after the initial appointment with the gynecologist, my worst fears were confirmed. On April 2, 2013, I—along with about 60,220 other Americans that year—was diagnosed with thyroid cancer. Despite the seemingly large number, I felt like a party of one. In the days following the news, my emotions ranged from complete denial to utter defiance. When friends and family checked in for updates, my response was a curt, "It's thyroid cancer." To make it personal and put the *"I have"* before the diagnosis would give it too much power. During my entire journey, it was as if the thyroid cancer was its own entity, a shadow that followed me but was never a part of my reality.

On the afternoon I was diagnosed, I remember coming home and being on the phone—for hours—trying to pretend that the events of the day were just a bad dream. I called everyone I could think of, even people that I hadn't spoken to in years. It was that day that I called an old friend with whom I had lost touch. She, too, had faced a cancer diagnosis, and I think my fingers instinctively knew to dial her number for comfort. Sadly, seven months after that phone call, she unexpectedly passed away. However, during those months she served as my confidant and mentor, and she would be an inspiration for me to be the same to others as time and my journey went on.

In an effort to educate myself and see what I was facing, I did something people who've just been diagnosed with cancer are advised against—I Googled my diagnosis. I feverishly scoured everything I could find on the Internet, from reputable websites to patient chat rooms. The wealth of information, coupled with the horror stories that I came across, made the reality that I was desperate to deny even scarier.

In the weeks that followed, I began to consult with head-and-neck surgeons who were likely candidates to perform the total thyroidectomy I would eventually undergo to remove the butterfly-shaped gland at the base of my neck. The endocrinologist's parting words to me began to make sense as I went from doctor to doctor and tried to decide on a surgeon—never feeling confident with my options or my own ability to make this life-changing decision.

After seeing three surgeons, the time had come to choose one. I made lists, I solicited opinions from friends and family, and I again read reviews on the Internet. The deciding factor came from a dear friend of mine whose brother-in-law, an endocrinologist, suggested that I go with the surgeon who would proactively remove lymph nodes in my neck, to give me the best chance of preventing a recurrence. I didn't know it then, but those two people helped me avoid the likelihood of another surgery down the line. For that insight, I can never properly express my gratitude to them both.

Once I'd decided on a surgeon, I scheduled my operation for early May. But again, deep denial and fear left me paralyzed. I had convinced myself that I would die in surgery or, at the very least, that the diagnosis was somehow incorrect and I would undergo a thyroidectomy for nothing. At the suggestion of worried friends, I rescheduled the surgery for a later date.

The words of the endocrinologist were truer now than ever before. What was it going to take to make me feel comfortable enough to move forward? I replayed the last few months over and over in my head. The diagnosis was real, and my fear was, too. I finally got to the point where I had to make a conscious choice to close this chapter—and the only way to do that was to commit to having surgery.

On June 17, 2013, I underwent a total thyroidectomy with central-neck dissection and lymph-node removal. When I awoke in the recovery room, my surgeon's kind face greeted me, and he told me the good news. He had removed my thyroid and six lymph nodes, and he noted that the nodes he took out looked clean. There was no evidence that the cancer had spread. I was no longer someone with a diagnosis of thyroid cancer, but rather a cancer survivor.

I saw my surgeon for a post-operative appointment about a week later. The pathology results had come back. Of the six nodes that had been removed, one showed signs that the cancer had spread. I immediately thought back to that conversation with my friend—and his brother-in-law's sage advice. I had done a little reading about undergoing a radioactive-iodine treatment to eliminate any remaining thyroid cancer cells or thyroid tissue as a follow-up procedure during my research phase. I was sure that was going to be the next step.

To my great surprise, my surgeon had a different plan. Since my most recent blood work indicated that my anti-thyroglobulin antibody level, which can be used to monitor for persistent or recurrent disease, was trending downward, he felt comfortable adopting a wait-and-see protocol. Should my levels plateau or increase, we would do a course of radioactive iodine. I left his office that day elated, and it marked the first time in many months that I was able to think of something other than cancer.

With my diagnosis behind me, it was time to return to living my life. Only this time, I was living life as a thyroid cancer survivor. I started right where I had left off, seeking a career path that was personally and professionally rewarding—and also one that would allow me to give back and share my story with other newly diagnosed thyroid cancer patients.

While it was certainly easier to think I could just return to life as I knew it, the truth was, I couldn't. I had added the most important job title to my resumé—thyroid cancer survivor—and it was the only role I cared deeply about. I decided this was the time to start a blog. Going through a thyroid cancer diagnosis taught me in six months what I had been trying to learn in my 26 years: how to find my voice. My first step was to start a blog on Word-press—a little space on the Internet that I called Living in Steil (pronounced style), to share my story.

From the beginning, my story as a survivor was prominently featured on my blog. When I was diagnosed, I didn't know anybody who'd had thyroid cancer, and I didn't know where to turn. I knew I probably wasn't alone in those feelings. I remembered how traumatic it was to read the less-than-op-timistic stories in the days after my diagnosis—stories like, "I started taking daily synthetic thyroid-hormone replacement medication, and I gained all this weight, and I feel terrible" or, "I had a thyroidectomy and I never felt the same."

I wanted to use my story to create a positive site and resource for people, a place where newly diagnosed patients could hear me say, "I had thyroid cancer. This is what happened. This is everything that I went through, and I'm OK. I made it to the other side." I wanted to be that ray of sunshine for these patients on their hardest days.

Although the site was a way for me to get my story out there, I never planned on becoming an advocate. I once knew a woman who volunteered her time for something she was passionate about, and I asked her what made her do it. Her answer surprised me. She said that you don't choose the cause; it chooses you. From being a thyroid cancer survivor, I became an advocate. I started raising awareness about the importance of going to your doctor for a neck check, having your thyroid levels checked when you go for routine blood work, and being vigilant about your health. Working with efforts like Thyroid Cancer Awareness Month in September and Thyroid Disease Awareness Month in January, I made it my mission on my blog to educate a larger audi-ence about the importance of thyroid health. If by my sharing my story and knowledge, one person's thyroid cancer can be diagnosed earlier, I've done my job. The greatest compliment I receive as a blogger is when somebody reaches out and says, "Wow, your story really inspired me" or "I saw something on your site and decided to become a blogger too." Knowing my words resonated and were a source of inspiration for others is the best feeling in the world.

My cathartic side-hustle soon turned into more than just a place to house my health journey. I expanded it into a lifestyle site, focused on things relating to fashion, food, fitness, health, and wellness, to appeal to a larger audience and other like-minded Millennials who may or may not have had cancer. Within a few months I had brands reaching out to me as an influenc-er. More importantly, my creative outlet launched a career for me that I never expected.

In 2018, I was fortunate enough to find a job as a social media and public relations manager for a pancreatic cancer foundation. After becoming more involved in the cancer space and interacting with patients and survivors with different cancers, I decided to take my career one step further and enroll in a Health Coach Training Program. As a survivor, I want to give back and work one-on-one with people who are struggling with an ailment and looking to embark on healthier lifestyle habits.

Six years post-surgery, I continue to be under the care of an endocrinologist. I have routine neck ultrasounds and regular blood work to ensure that my daily synthetic thyroid-hormone replacement dose remains at an effective level. Some hiccups along the way have brought to mind that my status as a survivor should never be taken for granted. While my scar is virtually undetectable now, its remnants serve as an important reminder of how fragile life can be. I was blessed to have the support of family, good friends, and an amazing team of doctors at NewYork-Presbyterian/Weill Cornell Medical Center. But it was the thorough examination conducted by my gynecologist that led to early detection and my diagnosis.

While I wouldn't wish it on anyone, ironically, I am grateful for my thyroid cancer diagnosis. Cancer was the scariest teacher I've ever had, but it taught me the most lasting lessons: It showed me that I am stronger than my struggles, revealed strengths I never knew I had, and directed me down a path I didn't even know existed.

The thing I most want to say to a thyroid cancer patient is this: You will come out on the other side, and you will be OK. You're going to be the same person, but you'll have a different outlook on life. Once you've faced a health crisis, you stop sweating the small stuff and realize that every day brings something to be grateful for. To know that your health can be taken away at a moment's notice has a way of putting life in perspective for you in an instant.

Lip-Synch for Your Life

. . . .

Name: Molly Young

Town: Baltimore, Maryland

Diagnosis: Breast cancer stage 2; invasive ductal carcinoma

Age at diagnosis: 29

Age now: 31

Editors' note: Molly was interviewed for this book while she was finishing active treatment, as her essay reflects. She has since finished and has returned to the work and joy of her singing—out loud.

I was just as shocked as everyone else around me when I was diagnosed with breast cancer at age 29. I had just had a physical, I had no recent family history of breast cancer, and I'm negative for BRCA-gene mutations. I had no experience with hospitals. I had never even broken a bone.

I'm a musician, kind of a "high notes for hire" mercenary. I consider myself very lucky to get to make music for a living, with a very supportive community of colleagues whom I also consider friends. At the time I found the lump, I was working as a voice and piano teacher all day and in rehearsal for Mozart's *Die Zauberflöte* all night, getting home at like 11 or midnight. I didn't do anything about the lump for a few weeks, mainly because I really wanted it to be a cyst. I was very fortunate to have signed up for health insurance as of January 1st, because on February 24th, I was diagnosed with cancer.

> BEST ADVICE: Finding ways to let your guard down a little bit and allow loved ones to be helpful is not only likely beneficial for you as a patient, but also something that people around you want and need. There's a learning curve to being the patient, and a big part of that is allowing your community to hold you up.

When I thought about what my life was going to look like through chemo and how I was going to deal with it, I knew I needed a distraction. Between Adriamycin, Cytoxan, Taxol, and Herceptin, I was going to have 30 infusion appointments over 14 months. I couldn't bear the idea of sitting in a chemo chair for hours every week with just a book or TV show; that wasn't going to be enough to take me out of the suddenly horrific existence I was living.

I was driving to or from one of my numerous appointments when

Kelly Clarkson's "What Doesn't Kill You Makes You Stronger" came on the radio. As I started going through the words in my head, I had the idea to use the song somehow in relation to my treatment. The drugs that would soon be pushed into my system, destroying my hair and my nails and so many other healthy parts of me in the hopes of killing off the invasive cancer cells, would be tough to endure—but would ultimately save my life.

Singing loudly in the chemo ward while other patients were sleeping or dealing with their own treatments—often more taxing or painful than my own—wasn't an option; and as my treatment went on, my voice developed a rasp, anyway. I wouldn't have wanted to record it. Lip-synching videos occurred to me as the perfect solution, and it served as both a silly distraction for me and an entertaining way for my friends and family all over the world to see for themselves that I was in good spirits and all right.

There are around 16 stations in my oncology ward, each separated by curtains, and a couple of private rooms. I'm very aware that I'm generally 20 to 30 years younger than anyone else there, and many people are having a rougher go of it than I am. I don't flounce in with my Ikea bags full of costumes but try to be as discreet as I can. When I film the videos, I always keep the curtain closed.

I started the project for survival. Physically, I knew I could get through my treatment. It would be awful, rough, terrible, but I would get through it. My mental and emotional health are the bigger challenges. Like other young patients, I'm at a time in life where my career and relationships and family aren't yet fully formed. With life already in flux, it's hard to handle an abrupt and unwelcome disruption.

When I got my diagnosis, one of my earliest worries was that all I would be to people going forward was "Cancer Girl." I'm very uncomfortable being pitied. The last thing I wanted was to be looked at constantly with sad puppy eyes, and be told to sit in the corner and drink tea under my prayer shawls. I just couldn't. I remember sitting with my parents and my older brother, and saying, "This is the pink cancer…. Everyone's going to send me pink things. I hate pink." I needed a way to take ownership of myself and my story, and to hold on to who I was before I got sick. I've always been someone who's looking for the next thing to laugh at. The idea that this experience would change that about me, or take that away from me, is almost worse than the idea of it killing me. If I'm going to get to live, then I should get to live as myself. I felt early on that having a sense of humor through this was going to be pretty crucial. My videos would be a method of self-care—to remind myself that my own playfulness and whimsy survived, despite everything that had been taken away from me.

The videos started off fairly simply. My only "costume" was wearing bright-red lipstick in every video. As I continued, my baldness gave me opportunities to get creative. The videos expanded in scope and vision to become a weekly event of ridiculousness. It's to the point where I walk into the chemo ward with bags of costumes and makeup, and my nurses always look forward to finding out what the song of the day will be.

I've chosen songs that could be some kind of power anthem or encouragement. Other times I've just chosen something silly—whatever might make people feel better and make them smile. From the beginning, I've shared the videos not just with friends and family, but also on patient pages—because I know that if anyone needs a smile, it's cancer patients. I thought they would be able to relate: "You're seeing me in this chair. You've probably been there too. You know what this is like, and isn't this silly that I'm doing this?"

The first three videos are very simple and short: Kelly Clarkson, Destiny's Child, and Christina Aguilera, all woman-power-anthem type stuff. I hadn't really figured out the ins and outs of the technology yet, and the app I started with only let me do a 10-second clip. I look back on those and think, "This is terrible." But I did learn. A friend commented recently, "Wow, the cinematography is getting more advanced." "Well, I had a year of practice," I told her. I actually now know iMovie, so now I guess I can put that on my résumé.

Then I started one-upping myself. Before my July 4th treatment, I thought, *Well, I have to do something holiday-themed.* So I did "Firework" by Katy Perry. By then I was bald and had to think, "What can I get to stick to my head? Not sparklers—I definitely can't have lit fireworks in an oncology ward." I ended up finding these pinwheels at Walmart and snapped off the handles, then used eyelash glue to get them to stick to my head. It took a lot of playing around with it with my roommate to get them to stay on and also spin. When we finally got it to work, I felt a rush of utter glee. I was bald, I had a pinwheel stuck to my head, and I might be dying. It was macabre, but I was making it silly.

If no one had liked the videos, I really wouldn't have cared. The night before an infusion, instead of focusing on how the treatment was going to make me feel like walking death, all I thought about was trying to get all my props together and making sure I had the right adhesive glue. I could have sat around and felt really sorry for myself for a long time. I do have days when that still happens, but this was something I consciously gave myself, to let me keep choosing positivity, keep angling myself towards something happier.

It catapulted from there. I started thinking of characters and costumes. To me, the best were the really silly mashups, like when I did "Papa Can You Hear Me" from *Yentl* as Princess Leia, so she's singing about Darth Vader. Or, for Thanksgiving, I sang, "Empty Chairs at Empty Tables" from *Les Misérables*—but as a turkey. So the turkey's talking about all his friends having died. For me, the name of the game for the past year has been what can make me laugh, what can make me not be depressed and terrified about being a cancer patient.

My bald head became an opportunity. There were days when I woke up and looked in the mirror and just felt like this strange Gollum person. Days I felt like I couldn't face going out in public. But then there were days where I thought, *Well, this is kind of a cool canvas. What do I do with it?* One of my favorite videos was the duet from *Annie*. I was Little Orphan Annie and bald Daddy Warbucks, side by side. I thought, *If I'm going to be bald, I definitely have to be Daddy Warbucks. I can't give up that opportunity.* I did a series painting my head like the planets; I painted my head as a watermelon and a jack-o'-lantern…. Instead of mourning the loss of my hair all the time, I tried to shift my perspective to, "I have this period of time where I'm going to be able to draw on my scalp. That's kind of neat. Most people don't get to do that."

Early on, I did receive all sorts of the dreaded pink-ribbon stuff as gifts. But as the videos started getting shared in social media, people found more personal ways to show their support. Wearing bold lipstick started because I cut off all my hair and felt the need to compensate. But it gave a friend of mine the idea to get people to wear red lipstick and share selfies on my chemo days, as a show of solidarity. It caught on and became a really cool movement. Someone else called me "Wonder Woman" (the movie was out that summer) and sent me a Wonder Woman onesie, which later became a costume for one of the videos. That kind of gift replaced the sad packages of tea and pink ribbons. Thanks to the videos, there was this huge shift to strength and power and encouragement, as opposed to pity and sorrow. That's something I really, really needed at the time and something I wanted. I had so little control over my body during treatment, but the videos gave me some control over the narrative and how people thought or talked about me.

Looking back, I can see that doing the videos also satisfied my performer psychology. I need to entertain people. That's something that I've done all my life and do for a living. Whether or not I could have verbalized it then, I felt the need to compensate for this darkness I had brought into everyone's lives. I needed to do something to make sure they knew it was going to be OK. I'm sure anyone reading this will say, "You're the patient! You need to be the one who is comforted!" But I couldn't help but worry about everyone else. I knew my mother would have done anything to switch places with me. (She's told me this roughly 38 times by now.) I have so many people in my support circles who are really far away and couldn't see me in person, to be comforted or relieved that I am still alive. The videos could be like a little postcard—me being like, "Hey, I'm still kicking. I'm going to fight this. This is not the end." I needed some way to prove that to them and give them something to think about besides me dying.

The extent to which my videos have been shared, or have affected other patients, has been a humbling surprise to me. I have received countless messages from friends, or friends of friends of friends, telling me how they or someone they loved was just diagnosed, is struggling through treatment, or is having a hard time—and they saw one of my videos, and it helped them smile that day. One message came from a patient whose daughter was four or five when she was first diagnosed. That's a really scary situation for a child. I had never thought about it from that angle because I don't have children, even though I interact with them a lot as a teacher. Kids have to watch their parents go through treatment, and seeing them sick and tired all the time is a lot to deal with. This woman wrote, "You've given my daughter another way to see cancer. She can see all the same equipment that mom uses but in this silly context. It's not trying to pretend that the cancer's not there or gloss over the experience, but it's making it something that she can also laugh at. That is such a powerful thing, and I'm really grateful."

That letter cut me right to the bone. I was like, "Oh, my gosh." The daughter even wrote me a Christmas card and said, "What would I do without you? You make me happy and not sad." I burst into tears when I read that. I'm a Harry Potter nerd. I started to see the videos like a Riddikulus charm, where you take whatever you're most afraid of and turn it into something that you can laugh at to destroy its power.

Now it's almost a year later and I have only two Herceptin infusions left, which means two more videos. I don't see myself continuing to make them when I'm done with treatment. But when Facebook started showing me "Memories" of my videos, I felt like I needed to communicate another layer of the experience, now that I have more distance. I wanted people to know that beyond the silly fun, there was another side to the story that was painful and terrifying. I was so scared. So for example, when I shared my very first video again, I added a note about the awful backstory—like how I hadn't have lidocaine yet that day, so I felt everything when the nurse put the needle into my chemo port, which really hurt.

As much as I still want to brighten people's days and make them smile and laugh, I think it's also valuable to bring a more honest lens to the experience. I'm far enough removed now that I can tell people, without them worrying I'm sitting there sobbing in that moment, that just because someone is posting selfies of themselves smiling, it doesn't mean everything is OK. Humor is as important as ever, but I also want to shine a light on the mental health of cancer patients. It's not just are we throwing up on the floor, are we sick, are we in pain, but where is our psyche? How are we feeling, just as people? I'm not comfortable with my videos existing alone as this inspiring, perfect, brave caricature of a cancer patient. I wouldn't ever want them to make a patient feel bad about herself if she's not as positive as I seem to be. I feel an obligation now to bring some awareness to the fact that cancer is a total mixed bag.

One thing I've had to learn along the way is no matter what, no matter how well any treatment goes or how responsive your body is, there's always a chance that somewhere down the road you could have a recurrence, that this could happen all over again, that it could spread somewhere else in your body. I recently watched a friend who was exactly my age with exactly my diagnosis progress to stage 4 and die within another four months. It's a shocking jolt back to reality—that this is not all fun and games and costumes, but real people actually die. I could be one of those people. That's absolutely a sobering reality check.

Now that my treatment is ending, managing the anxiety of what will happen or when it will happen is a new challenge. 30% of early-stage patients (which I am) become late-stage patients, but that means that 70% do not. I could very well live to be 70 or 80, and I don't want to use the rest of that time constantly looking over my shoulder. On my best days, I can see the anxiety as a positive; it encourages me to experience life and joy a little more authentically.

This year I experienced the blossoming in the spring and the turn of the seasons as a hugely poignant landmark; last spring I was still getting scanned, still getting cut open, still feeling like someone's science experiment. Life is just super short, and it's shorter now than I knew it to be a year ago. As a result, I've been more attentive to carving out personal time, getting outside more, doing more hiking, doing the things that complete me as a person. I hope that will be one lasting change in my outlook.

Acknowledgments

This book was funded on Kickstarter.

TOUGH was made possible because of those named below and many others who chose to remain unnamed.

Thank you all from the bottom of my heart. - Marquina

Patti & Simeon Iliev

Dan Piselli

Benjamin Iliev

Bianka Iliev

Aimee Fearon

Amy Reynolds

Andrea Griffiths

Angela Zallen

Ann & Frank Chiarello

Ann E Freedman

Barbara Muller Bowen

Beth Cooperstein

Beverly Schley

Brad & Stacy Delaney

Casey & Caroline Fatchett

Christopher, Paige & Rowan Sealey

Colleen M. Greer

Colleen Newvine Tebeau

Conor Sullivan

Constance Stangarone

David Mayseless

Dolly Kelly

Dr. Justin Dugas

Dugas Dental - Family & Cosmetic Dentistry

Elaine Corona

Elana Schwam

Elena Contreras Gullickson

Eletra M Johansen

Emily Strong

Erica Frenkel

Erica Heinz

Erin Nicole Brown Photography

Eva (the Diva) Newborn

Evelina Gokinayeva

Foli Ayivoh

Gentile/Birardi Family

Headliner Video

Jaime Siskosky

Jamie Hitchings

Janet Chambers

Janie Yamato

Jeff Moore

Jenna Gibson

Jennifer Bol

Jessica Harris

Jim Lane

Joe & Michelle LeVine

John M Copic

Kate Minckler

Kathryn Hust

Kelly Gonsalves

Kylene Griffith Terhune

Laura deNey

Lia Fioroni

Lizzy Gannon Mack

LJ Porter

Masayo K

Matthew Wilkins

Michael Kovnat

Mike and Tami Langenright

Mindy Buchanan

MJ Babic

Neil Baptista

Nicholas Sheets

Nichole Wouters

Pauline L. Mercer

Rachael Vaughn

Rachel "Agnes Young" Sinclair

Rachel Jensen

Rebecca Krav

Robin Glazer

San Diego Air Guitar

Sara MacKimmie

Sarah Canner

Sarah Dickman

Scott Bowman

Shala Nicely

Smo

Sonya Davis

Stephanie Cox-Connolly

Sue Ellen Schwam

Tom Wolan

Tory Messina

Trish Brennan

Vincent Fung

Made in United States
North Haven, CT
11 July 2022

21206284R00125